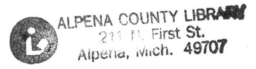

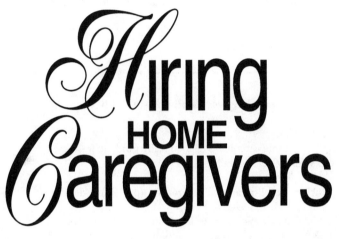

Hiring HOME Caregivers

The Family Guide to In-Home Eldercare

649.8
SUSI
(v)

D. Helen Susik, M.A.

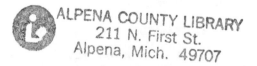
American Source Books
A DIVISION OF
Impact Publishers®, Inc.
SAN LUIS OBISPO, CALIFORNIA

Library of Congress Cataloging-in-Publication Data

Susik, D. Helen.
    Hiring home caregivers : the family guide to in-home
eldercare / D. Helen Susik.
        p.   cm.
    Includes bibliographical references (p.   ) and index.
    ISBN: 0-915166-91-7
    1. Aged--Home care. 2. Domestics. 3. Caregivers.
4. Visiting housekeepers. 5. Home health aides.   I. Title.
HV1451.S77   1995
649.8'068'3--dc20   94-46163
                                                                    CIP

Printed in the United States of America on acid-free paper
Cover design by Sharon Schnare, San Luis Obispo, California
Author photo by John P. Lofreddo, University of South Florida, Health
    Sciences Media Center

Published by **American Source Books**
A DIVISION OF
Impact Publishers,® Inc.
POST OFFICE BOX 1094
SAN LUIS OBISPO, CALIFORNIA 93406

Contents

For Memaw

HELEN FLORA BAKER HAMBRICK

1888 - 1971

ACKNOWLEDGEMENTS

I OWE THANKS TO THOSE INTERESTED IN OLDER PEOPLE AND the quality of their lives who have helped me, especially Janice Blanchard, Eugenia Williamson and Lynn Friss for manuscript review; Edith Freedman for encouragement and support; Mary Brooks, for setting an inspiring example; Bill Corristan and Mike Hinson for tax advice; Marian Wingo and Chris Vinsonhaler, for sisterly encouragement and Emmanuel Martin, for shared professional contacts. A special debt of gratitude is due my husband, M.B. Susik, a human resources professional who guided me through the shoals of the book's latter chapters, and Pat Geasa, who helped every day.

Other technical expertise on bonding was contributed by Sharon Daugherty of Sevitex; on background investigations by Tom Halliburton of Global Investigations and Information Network; and on criminal investigations by Ed Geasa of the Hillsborough County, Florida, S.A.L.T. Council (Seniors and Law Enforcement Officers Together.)

I was privileged to receive manuscript critique from a team of top-level aging service professionals from across the nation. Their names and areas of specialization are listed in the book's end pages.

My final thanks must go to my beloved daughter, Abigail, for sharing me with the demands of writing, to Steven Phillips, founder of American Source Books, without whose vision and guidance this book could never have been written, and to Deborah McPherson, for professional secretarial support.

PREFACE

MEN AND WOMEN AGED ABOUT SEVENTY-FIVE AND OLDER face enormous challenges. What if arthritis gets so bad that bathing or dressing without help becomes impossible? What if fading eyesight makes driving to the grocery store too dangerous? Or if a cane, walker or wheelchair makes cooking meals and cleaning the house a slow and painful ordeal?

These are the facts of life for millions across America today. Every year, more and more older people look to someone else for help with the simple yet crucial things: washing and dressing, cooking and housecleaning, shopping and driving. More than eight million older Americans need assistance with personal care.

This trend will only intensify as we live longer than ever before, in a world of increasing complexity. In fact, providing care for older loved ones represents a growing national crisis that will touch nearly every American family.

Living Longer, Living Better

The good news is, not only are we living longer, we are living better. Our world is literally exploding with products and services designed to help maintain independence throughout the life span. Of course, a major emphasis today is on keeping men and women at home and out of nursing homes. Thus, home care is the fastest-growing segment of the health care industry.

In the race to develop programs to help families and elders, an interesting thing has happened, however. Service providers have assumed many responsibilities that until recently were managed by families. Elders are often classified as "cases," whose care requires "management" by medical experts. The assumption that "eldercare" means "medical care" represents an over-reaction to the challenges of long-term care. Older persons are most often not "patients"; they are simply older versions of the productive men and women they've always been. They don't want to be managed; they want a little extra help so that they can continue managing by themselves.

Consumer-driven Homecare?

Surprisingly, little has been written to help elders and families who need help in their efforts to manage independently. This book fills that gap by offering detailed guidance on *consumer-driven home care*. This approach allows the family to rely mainly upon its own resources (family members themselves, friends, neighbors, community), but reinforces this network with an in-home employee. Termed a "home caregiver," the employee is hired, supervised, and paid directly by the elder and family. Self-reliance is the core of this approach to home care.

What's the Advantage for Elders and Families?

Why would anyone choose to sidestep the wealth of formal home care services that are presently available? Consumers cite several compelling reasons. First, it's hard to deny that the person who directly recruits, supervises and pays an employee is truly in the driver's seat. Consumers have much to gain in terms of quality and control. This is the option for those intent on having things done the right way — theirs.

Second, although not all the research is in, results generally support the self-directed model as a cost-effective approach. Because elders may have limited financial resources to pay for home care and typically require from five to seven years of service, costs are a very significant issue when it comes to planning for the "third/third" of life.

Finally, when hiring a worker directly, loyalties and responsibilities lie solidly with the consumer-employer. This cuts out the middle-man, and along with it, a lot of bureaucratic preoccupations (service quotas, profit margins, regulatory realities, etc.). Instead, the main focus is upon a personal relationship with a real human being. In such a scenario, elders may have more of an opportunity to find what they need most — simple human caring.

A Few Notes on Style

The term "elder" is used throughout this book to denote older adults in their seventies, eighties and nineties — those at the oldest end of the age continuum. As all persons are unique, it is both difficult and unwise to make generalizations based on age. The idea is, however, that with advanced years, the need for personal assistance usually increases.

"Home caregiver" (or at times, "home helper") is used in this book to identify those who assist elders with their daily routine. Care may be given in a variety of settings, from private homes, to apartments, to shared living arrangements. In some cases, the help may focus on light housekeeping; in other cases, care might be limited to personal care or supervision. Suffice it to say that "home caregivers" are *those who provide the paid, non-medical support to help maintain well-being, personal appearance, comfort and safety.*

The term "family," which appears here almost as often as "elder" and "home caregiver," designates those who are related to one another through blood or marriage, as well as those who care for one another as a result of a long-term personal commitment. When it comes to hiring arrangements, the participation of a highly involved family member is recommended, and assumed here.

The pronoun "she" is used in this book when referring to caregivers because the vast majority of those who provide care to elders are women. "She" is also used when referring to elders themselves. Given the fact that longevity is greater for females, most of those on the receiving end of care are also women.

Sources of Information

Information on hiring caregivers has been gleaned in part from the independent living movement. Hiring home helpers is routine for disabled adults, and much of what has been learned by this population applies nicely to the elderly.

Home care agencies have provided another rich source. Agencies have amassed a wealth of practical information based on experience. "Trade secrets" were unearthed in the industry literature, in policy and personal manuals, and through personal interviews with administrators, supervisors and front-line staff.

A number of states now have centers established specifically to help and support family caregivers. For example, California's statewide system of Caregiver Resource Centers offers a direct pay option where families can hire their own home helpers. The approach discussed here has much in common with many of these progressive projects.

Organizations such as the American Association of Retired Persons (AARP) have supplied consumer-oriented pamphlets and publications — free for the asking. Several such organizations, which can be of considerable help to those pursuing homecare, are listed at the end of each chapter.

Perhaps the most valuable lessons have been learned from elders themselves, and their families. Some have shared success stories; others stories of frustration and failure. These shared experiences provide us an opportunity to profit from the real-life experiences of others. You'll find some of their stories in the pages that follow.

A Final Word . . .

This book will have its critics. Some will say that the consumer-directed approach is old fashioned and home-spun, placing insufficient weight upon quality control, health and safety issues and legal protections for both the consumer and the home care worker. This is just another way of saying that elders and families are not competent to manage their own care. Certainly, consumer-directed eldercare involves a balancing act between choice and control on the one hand, and managed risks on the other.

Some may be uncomfortable with this book's bottom-line message: "Don't be passive! Take charge of the whos, hows, whens and wheres of home care! You can do it!" But, of course, not all families wish to accept the responsibilities of self-managed care, and not all families have the capacity to do so.

It's critically important to stress the point that the consumer-directed option is not for everyone. Many of the managerial functions of self-directed home care, such as paying employment taxes and conducting background checks, are unavoidably tedious and time-consuming. Asking some families to shoulder these tasks, in addition to their already heavy physical and emotional burdens of eldercare, is simply unrealistic.

It is also important to emphasize that a "mixed-mode" approach is the most desirable. In other words, independent hiring is just one of the many options that elders and families should have at their disposal when seeking to construct a plan for care over the long term. Perhaps the most durable plans represent an interface of professional and family resources.

Care can be a bit like a jigsaw puzzle. Hiring home caregivers represents only a single piece of the puzzle — one that may or may not fit for a given family. Meeting the challenge of caring requires the creativity of fitting many pieces together: family involvement, formal agency services, hired helpers, friends and neighbors, religious and community resources, volunteers and other options.

Finally, relying on in-home help may represent only a short-term solution. For many, the time will come when round-the-clock care or skilled, health-related services are needed. Elders and families must plan ahead by researching other options, including relocation to a more supportive setting, or skilled nursing care. Knowing when the time has come to increase levels of support is part of the challenge of home care, and one this book will help you recognize.

— *D. Helen Susik*
February 1995

Chapter One

YOU'RE THE BOSS!

"I hate to say it, but I'm getting to be so 'no count' that getting out of bed and getting ready to face the world each day, is fast becoming a problem for me. I hate housework and cooking, and sometimes I'd rather skip a meal than go to a cafe to get it. It isn't that I don't have the money, or that I hate to spend it, it's just old age, I would say. But I better not knock that — I may have quite a few years ahead, and hope I do."

— R. Ewing, age 87

WHAT DO ELDERS WANT? THEY WANT TO HOLD ON TO AS much health and independence as possible, without posing an undue burden to their families or to society. They want to feel safe, informed and in control of the decisions in their lives. Perhaps most of all, they wish to live out their days in that setting that is preferable to all others: *their own homes.*

Mr. Ewing could certainly benefit from hiring a home caregiver. In fact his family is probably urging him to hire someone to help him manage around the house — a caring, dependable person who could function almost as a loving relative. She would see that his house is clean, and that he is comfortable, well-fed and well-cared for in general. Sounds like a great idea, doesn't it?

The need for personal assistance with daily living is a fact of life for millions of Americans. For many, assistance with personal care and housework is necessary for survival. With adequate assistance, many elders like Mr. Ewing can continue with an independent lifestyle, aging with dignity within their homes and communities. Without it, they may find themselves increasingly threatened by a move to a long term care facility.

What in the World Is a Home Caregiver?

In the U.S.A., we have not yet arrived at a standard term for workers who attend to the practical needs of elders at home. "Home helper" is the term used in Scandinavian countries. Since "home care" has become a widely recognized term for the *process* of providing in-home help, "home caregiver" has been selected as the descriptive term to be used in this book.

Home caregivers help elders with eating, grooming and dressing. They give baths and brush dentures. They escort to the bathroom and change soiled linen. They may be expected to straighten the house, wash dishes and do the laundry. When an elder needs non-medical help at home, the home caregiver is often the best choice for a busy family.

Of course, people of all ages and abilities sometimes must rely upon another person to meet their daily needs. For example, a home helper for children might be called a *nanny*, for a disabled adult a *personal care attendant*, and for a Medicare recipient, a *homemaker/home health aide*.

Scope of the Book

The world of home care is bursting with service options and service models. This book deals with only one: *consumer-directed home care*. In this model, the employee works neither for herself nor for a nonprofit or profit-making agency. She works for the consumer, in a direct employer/employee relationship. In this consumer-directed approach, elders and families take full responsibility for managing their own program of in-home care. The consumer is The Boss.

Hiring Home Caregivers covers only employment arrangements for part-time or full-time home caregivers, as opposed to 24-hour *live-in* assistance. Live-in arrangements comprise a unique and separate category for tax purposes, and really deserve special treatment in a separate publication.

The book limits its discussion to *non-medical personal care* services. The home caregiver discussed here will not be nurse-supervised; neither will she be guided by a medical doctor's plan of treatment. She will be a non-professional, unskilled or semi-skilled worker who may be untrained, or may be a graduate of a vocational or trade school.

Hiring Home Caregivers is not about skilled nursing care or high tech medical services; it is about assistance that can help an elder continue living at home.

Overview of the Book

Chapter 2 explains the various tasks of in-home helpers, differentiates between home-helpers and medical workers and discusses costs and sources of financial assistance.

Chapter 3 provides checklists to aid in decision-making. The reader will gain a clearer understanding about when — in terms of health and financial abilities — hiring independently represents a viable option, and when it may be more appropriate to move on to more professional or health-oriented services. The reader will also be introduced to two professional services that can aid in planning for long term care: M.D. geriatric practitioners and geriatric care managers.

Chapters 4 through 7 lay out the nuts and bolts of writing ads, developing job descriptions, screening, interviewing and negotiating employment agreements. You will learn how to assure that duties are specifically assigned and mutually understood.

Chapter 8 takes you beyond hiring and gives you the basics of open, honest and direct communication techniques (how to offer constructive praise and criticism, and how to supervise the home caregiver once she is hired).

Chapter 9 introduces the reader to the world of aging services, or those home- and community-based programs designed to help elders maintain their independence.

Chapter 10 provides indispensable guidance and management tools for paying necessary taxes, social security and insurance.

The final chapter lays out the agency-directed option of home care/home health care that can supplement or eventually replace your own program of consumer-directed eldercare.

This book was written to give readers the "know how" to begin and end home care for elders. For readers who have never considered hiring and supervising on their own, the book will answer the question "How do I start?" For more experienced employers, it can fine-tune background checking, tax management, record-keeping and other administrative skills.

Specifically, readers of *Hiring Home Caregivers* will learn to:
- recruit home helpers
- screen applicants
- conduct interviews — telephone and face-to-face
- check references
- check public records
- write an employment agreement
- set work schedules
- train and evaluate
- pay wages and taxes
- maintain records
- dismiss when necessary
- access home- and community-based service

- use agency services to supplement consumer-directed home care.

What this Book Can Do for You

In-home personal assistance as an answer to the challenge of caring for an older adult is wonderful in theory, but complicated in real life. We no longer live in a world where a neighbor down the street will be delighted to look in on an aging loved one as a favor — or even in return for a little spending money. Today, the neighbor very likely holds down a full-time job and those who might be interested in working as a home caregiver expect to make at least minimum wage. And if we intend to hire someone we have some very specific responsibilities — to ourselves, to those we hire and to Uncle Sam.

No one is born a personnel manager. Most Americans don't have experience in recruiting, interviewing, setting wages or negotiating agreements. They may know nothing of employer taxes and liability issues. But with good information, these skills can be learned, and that's why this book was written.

If you decide to give the consumer-driven approach a try, this book will help you meet the challenge. You will learn how to advertise, how to interview, how to negotiate and how to make sure that your home helper is safe, healthy, and dependable. You will learn how to pay taxes, file records and stay on the good side of Uncle Sam. You will gain access to information that would take hours to amass on your own: labor law, personnel management, bookkeeping, insurance and other issues.

In addition to all that, with any luck at all, you may find that caring person who will brighten your days, lighten your burdens, and touch your heart. Is that really too much to ask when it comes to living longer and living better?

Chapter Two

THE ROLE AND COST
OF HOME CAREGIVERS

"Poor mother has been burned on her forearms, often badly, while cooking. We also suspect she is not eating right, judging by the stash of frozen meat pies that she keeps on hand.

Mother cannot shampoo her long hair nor get out of the tub without help. She has slipped and fallen recently in the bathtub. She cannot zip her dress, and this embarrasses her a great deal. Just last week my brother whispered , 'What on earth are we going to do about mother?' "

— Fiona Baker, age 61, employed caregiver

THE ADULT WHO LIVES ALONE BUT DOESN'T EAT RIGHT, SLIPS in the tub, leaves the stove on, neglects to pay the bills, or wanders and becomes lost needs help from her family. She also may need extra in-home help to avoid being moved to a more restrictive (institutional) setting.

Most of us have a good understanding of the role doctors, nurses, and other professionals could play in helping someone like Mrs. Baker's mother, who is beginning to have trouble managing the ordinary activities of daily living. The role of home helper is much less clearly understood, however. That's because this job is a new and developing one.

A home caregiver is a paid employee who assists with personal care, household tasks and perhaps transportation. The job can be part-time or full-time and usually pays slightly more than minimum wage. Four hours of work per day is about standard; but the daily time worked depends primarily upon the needs of the elder.

Paid care for elders was almost unheard of in years past. Help at home was usually provided by wives, daughters and daughters-in-law. This tested, tried and true caregiving was mostly about creating a comfortable old age. It had almost nothing to do with doctors, nurses, hospitals or nursing homes.

The old-fashioned form of caregiving is also the newest; and the demand for this basic care is reaching epic proportions. Today, this type of care is referred to as long-term care, maintenance care, or even "low-tech" care. Now that women are likely to be occupied at the workplace, and families often live at a distance from one another, reinforcement on the home-front is needed. Although most care is still provided by family members, paid home care is here to stay. Here are some of the reasons:

- preserves independence
- saves money
- prevents or postpones institutionalization
- provides maximum freedom
- improves the quality of life

What Do Home Helpers Do?
Hands-on Care

The provision of personal care, or "hands-on care" is the defining feature of a home caregiver's job. This clearly distinguishes her job from that of a maid or domestic servant. Rather than care of the home, her greater concern is care of the person:

- bathing/shampooing

- brushing hair
- brushing teeth
- make-up/care of skin (unbroken)
- shaving
- dressing
- toileting
- feeding

Light Housekeeping

Housekeeping is referred to as "light" because it is incidental to direct personal care of the elder. Home caregivers don't wash windows, do yard work, heavy chores, or serve an entire family. They do perform many duties for the elder that are indirectly related to personal care:

- personal laundry
- vacuuming
- meal preparation
- tidying rooms
- dishwashing
- changing linens

Supervision

Because the home caregiver does not work under the supervision of a doctor or a nurse, she limits herself to non-medical tasks, such as:

- preparing special meals (low fat or sodium)
- maintaining hygiene
- monitoring health status
- assisting with self-administered medications

Assisting with Mobility

The home caregiver assists the elder in moving from one place to another; for instance, to get into the bathroom or in and out of bed. Sometimes this involves help to and from the following:

- bed to wheelchair

- bed to commode
- wheelchair to walker
- walker to chair

The home caregiver assists the elder to follow a self-administered therapy program as prescribed by a licensed therapist. As mentioned above, she may also assist the elder with any braces or assistive devices, after instruction.

Companionship

A home caregiver can be a vital source of moral support to an elder who is beginning to lose independence, social contacts, and interactions with the community.

The home caregiver enhances the quality of life for the elder through:

- reading
- music
- walks
- letter writing
- conversation
- assisting with interests

Transporting and Escorting

Lack of adequate transportation is one of the main problems facing elders who are struggling to live independently. Some have never learned to drive, while others have had to give up driving due to health problems. A home caregiver who drives can run errands and take the elder to appointments.

The home caregiver might do the driving herself, or provide escort on public transportation for:

- shopping
- visiting
- eating out
- doctor and dental appointments
- banking
- post office

- pharmacy

In addition to the tasks outlined above, home caregivers who develop close relationships with an elder and family will often do the extras. When questioned about what their home caregivers do for them, elders frequently mention things like the following:

- "Calls to check between visits."
- "Sits down and talks a bit."
- "Will pick up medicine for me."
- "Brings a little joke each day."
- "Always asks me how I am and then sits quietly while I talk."

Special Tasks for Home Caregivers
Medications

A home caregiver *assists* with oral medications, rather than administering them herself. State nursing practice acts generally prohibit unlicensed workers from handing over medications, or measuring them out. This means the caregiver can arrange the medicine so it's convenient, bring a glass of water, remind when it's time, and stand by to watch that it's taken at the right dose.

A medication check-off chart is often helpful to make sure that medications are taken at the correct time. Check-offs are made when each medication is taken. (A sample chart is found at the end of this chapter.) Or pre-measured medications can be purchased at a pharmacy, as can plastic containers with compartments that are useful for pre-arranging each day's dosages.

Families should make sure to explain all aspects of the medicine regimen to the home caregiver, including:

- name of medicine
- purpose of the medicine
- color and shape of medicine

- correct dosage
- when to take the medicine
- how to take the medicine
- side effects
- renewable or not
- pharmacy name and phone number

The home caregiver should be instructed to communicate any questions, concerns or changes noted relating to medications to the family right away. She should also be given the names and phone numbers of the elder's physician and pharmacist. A home caregiver should not administer even over-the-counter medications without prior permission from a responsible family member.

Injections

If the elder is a diabetic, daily insulin injections may be required. This can usually be handled by the elder or a family member who is trained and experienced in this procedure. It is important to remember that injections are considered skilled nursing care, requiring the services of a RN or LPN. The home caregiver can fill the syringe and hand it to the elder at the prescribed time, but she shouldn't give the injection herself.

Bowel and Bladder Care

Some elders may have lost control of bowel or bladder, necessitating the use of absorbency products for incontinence. The home caregiver can help with a toileting regimen, and can change adult diapers as needed. (When involved in any procedure involving body fluids, the home caregiver should wear protective latex gloves to prevent the spread of infectious diseases.)

Other elders may need assistance with catheter or colostomy bags. The home helper can empty bags and dispose of wastes, but again, gloves should always be worn when performing these tasks.

Transportation

If a home caregiver will be transporting the elder by car, take a test drive with her. Pay attention to how she handles the car, her attitude toward other drivers, and willingness to accommodate your wishes. It is important that you consider all of these points since the elder's safety and peace of mind will completely depend on the driver.

For information on insurance coverage in this situation, see Chapter 7.

Emergencies

Be sure to let the home caregiver know of any emergency situations that have occurred in the past, or that might occur in the future. Post your doctor's name and number in a handy place, such as inside a cupboard door. Place the local number for reporting emergencies directly on the telephone. Use the forms "Emergency Telephone Numbers" and "Elder Information Form" at the end of Chapter 8.

Handling Money

Home caregivers need money to purchase food, supplies, prescription medications and other items. Caregivers may also need to cash checks and pay bills. Specific rules must be communicated regarding:

- written receipts
- returning change
- saving receipts and sales tags
- using identification cards and check cashing cards

Shopping

Plan a shopping trip in a way that insures that the correct items will be purchased. Make a shopping list that specifies preferred brands and quantities. Some families use a system whereby a separate purse, which contains family money is used by the home helper. Money designated for shopping is kept here, as are change and receipts.

If the elder is on a special diet, (low salt, low sugar, low fat) the home helper may need some extra instructions on reading labels as one aspect of her grocery shopping duties.

Paramedical Services

Some elders will have care needs that are not clearly medical in nature, but are generally considered to require licensed nursing supervision. Special bowel and bladder care, tube feeding and insulin injections fall into this *paramedical* category.

States regulate the delivery of skilled nursing and paramedical services through "nurse practices acts," which vary from state to state. Most typically preclude anyone other than family members and/or licensed professionals from performing nursing functions. This type of legislation clearly excludes home helpers.

Some states, like California, are more liberal, allowing the performance of nursing/paramedical functions by any person as long as a physician orders it and the person does not "in any way assume to practice as a professional, registered graduate or trained nurse." Caution, discretion and sound judgment are the points to remember in regard to unlicensed individuals, state restrictions and performance of paramedical functions.

Home caregivers should *never* be expected or required to provide care that is clearly medical in nature, such as wound care or ventilator service. For further clarification on these issues, contact your State Board of Nursing for a copy of its nurse practices act. This act, which is different in every state, outlines the rules and regulations that apply to medical versus non-medical patient care practices.

Health Monitoring

It is extremely important for the home caregiver to immediately notify the family about any change in the elder's health; for example, if the elder is not eating, is having pain, or seems in any way uncomfortable or changed.

Because the home caregiver may have more contact with the elder than do family members, these reports may be crucial to assuring the elder's safety and comfort.

On a more routine basis, the home caregiver can assist the elder with the self-monitoring of temperature, pulse, blood pressure and weight. She can observe, record and report self-administered medications (see medications charts at the end of this chapter). The caregiver can play a vitally important role in health monitoring by encouraging compliance with special diets and/or prescribed physical exercise routines.

What Home Caregivers Shouldn't Do
- administer medications
- irrigate the bladder
- insert medical devices (such as catheters, enemas, suppositories)
- change dressings (wound care)
- clip toenails
- monitor high-tech medical equipment
- provide active therapy
- other activities requiring judgment based on training given to licensed health care professionals

How Much Should You Pay for Your Caregiver?
As of this writing, federal law requires that you pay a home caregiver at least $4.25 an hour (current minimum wage). You must also pay Social Security benefits. Remember that wages have gone up with inflation over the last few years. If you offer too little in wages, you may be unable to get reliable help.

Using the minimum wage as the starting point, here are some other considerations in "how much to pay":
- the cost of living in your area of the country
- a comparison to what agencies are charging for comparable services

• benefits that you elect to provide

What Do Agencies Charge?

Perhaps the first step in answering the question of how much to pay is to check with several home care agencies to learn the going rate for services. Medicare-certified agencies usually have multiple sources of reimbursement for their services: Medicare, other third-party payors and/or out-of-pocket payment directly from customers. You are interested in the out-of-pocket part of their business. So, when you call to inquire, ask to be connected with the department that handles *private pay* services, as opposed to Medicare/Medicaid services.

Home health aide
(bathing, toileting, feeding and dressing)
Wage: $13/hour*

Homemakers
(household chores such as cleaning, cooking and shopping)
Wage: $9.50/hour

Companions/Sitters
(attend to the elder without much hands-on care)
$8.50 to $12/hour

Live-In Companion$90 to $125/day
Wage: $90 to $125/day

Fees listed are average charges in Tampa, Florida, 1995

Charges are generally higher in large cities, lower in small towns. Charges tend to be higher in the Northeast and West Coast, and lower in the South.

It's also important to realize that agencies in a single city will charge different prices for the same type of services. This means that, if you call to compare prices, you can save up to several dollars on a single hour of service. Additionally, some agencies won't send a worker out for less than three or four hours at a time. That averages out to about $40 per three-hour visit.

Does Insurance Pay for Home Care?

Private insurances, federal programs and state subsidies will sometimes cover a portion of the cost of home care, if eligibility is met and restrictions don't apply. These arrangements usually require working through a certified home health agency, rather than hiring independently. Reimbursement options are reviewed here in order to help you understand your alternatives in terms of financing home care.

Medicare pays for in-home help only in very specific circumstances, and for limited periods of time when:
- elder is confined to home by illness or injury
- elder needs part-time, *skilled* health care
- elder is under the care of a physician, who has ordered home health care service.

If an elder meets these criteria, Medicare will pay for personal care and housekeeping services in conjunction with skilled medical services. A beneficiary typically receives about one hour of care a day from two to five times a week. Services must be provided by a Medicare-certified home health agency and generally end after about six to eight weeks.

Medicaid is being used more and more often by states to pay for basic in-home care. If your relative has a very limited income, she may be eligible for this joint federal/state program. (In many states, people with higher incomes can qualify for Medicaid if they have high medical expenses.) Contact your local department of social services, public assistance or Area Agency on Aging office for further information.

Private health insurance policies (long term care insurance) now provide partial coverage for certain health-related home care services. Policies often have rules limiting in-home coverage, however, such as requiring prior hospitalization. Check individual insurance policies to see what may be covered, or contact the insurer. Most beneficial are the policies that pay for basic, personal care and housekeeping assistance.

Health Maintenance Organizations (HMOs) or prepaid group health plans often include some aspects of home care that provide funds to get clients out of expensive hospital settings. Check your individual managed care plan.

For now, reimbursement for unskilled home care is limited and restricted.

The bottom line is that much of the cost is not paid by governmental programs or private insurance policies. This means the money comes directly out of your family's personal budget. So, whether you are recruiting home caregivers yourself, or going through an agency, it can get expensive.

Do Public Programs Pay for Home Caregivers?

As of late 1994, home care is provided under at least nine federal authorities. Some provisions for home care services can be found, in addition to Medicare and Medicaid, in:

Older Americans' Act. OAA programs provide home-delivered meals, some in-home assistance (such as chore or homemaker), transportation and adult day care. Unlike Medicaid, the OAA serves persons aged 60+ of any income level. It must, however, target care to persons with greatest social or economic need. Contact an Area Agency on Aging (AAA) in your locale for further information.

The Veteran's Aide and Attendant Allowance. This allowance applies to eligible disabled veterans only. Veteran's benefits enable individuals to hire and manage their own home helpers. Contact the Department of Veteran Affairs.

Social Services Block Grant. SSBG funds also support a limited degree of in-home services for older persons. Thirty-five states use SSBG funds to provide homemaker/home health services. The SSBG does not require services to be provided only to persons with low incomes, but in practice most states direct these funds to low-income populations. Contact your state unit on aging or local AAA for further information.

Beneficiaries of Medicare, Medicaid and other federal programs, if they happen to live in communities with good Older Americans Act services, can often piece together a home care package that enables them to remain at home.

For further information about the Older Americans' Act and other federal programs, check the appendix. It should be noted that public programs are often limited in scope, restricted in eligibility, and can have waiting lists of up to two years.

Additionally, state, county and local governments offer a patchwork of special programs related to senior services and to home care. These programs often, but not always, service only those who meet certain income, health or social requirements. Some states (California, Massachusetts) have innovative programs that help elders and families locate home helpers and manage them through the consumer-directed approach discussed in this book. Check with the Department of Social Services in your state.

How Much Can You Save by Hiring Directly?

If you hire independently, you can generally expect to save about 30% "or more" off agency fees. Agencies must charge higher prices to cover rent, office overhead, worker's compensation, health benefits and general liability insurance.

The average hourly differential between an agency's reimbursement rate and wages paid to home caregivers represents an almost 100 percent markup for every hour of service. In other words, an agency-employed worker gets to keep only about half of the fees actually paid to an agency. The rest goes to overhead and profit.

In Florida, people hiring home caregivers independently are now (1995) paying about $6-$8 per hour for basic personal care. This represents a significant savings over the going agency rate of about $12 and up for the same service. Keep in mind, however, that you must add the cost of Social Security and other taxes when you hire directly; agencies include these costs in their fees.

Training for Home Caregivers

Workers in Medicare-certified home health agencies complete RN-supervised training, and pass a series of on-the-job and written tests. Understanding training requirements partially explains why agency fees are higher.

Home health aides are required to have at least 75 hours of classroom and supervised practical training in personal hygiene and grooming, safe transfer techniques, reading vital signs and ambulation. Trainees must then pass a final performance evaluation and a written or oral exam.

If you would like your independently-hired home caregiver to meet Medicare standards, you may wish to enroll her in a course of study. Training programs are typically offered by home health agencies, junior colleges and vocational and trade

schools. Training resource information can be found in
Appendix G.

Chapter 2 has introduced you to what home caregivers do
and how much their services cost. You've heard that home care
is the wave of the future, that it's one answer to keeping elders
out of nursing homes. Yet, the prices charged by home care
agencies are at a level that many of us simply cannot afford to
pay. After considering what private, state and federal
resources are available, you may decide that your best option
is hiring your own worker.

The viability of such a plan will depend upon your skill in
finding and managing personnel, and in handling paperwork
and keeping records. And it will most certainly depend upon
the elder's needs and resources, which will be discussed in the
next chapter.

MEDICINE CALENDAR			
Morning	Afternoon	Early Evening	Bedtime
Sun.			
Mon.			
Tues.			
Wed.			
Thurs.			
Fri.			
Sat.			

PRESCRIPTION MEDICINES

Date	Medicine	What for	Directions/Cautions	Prescribed by	End Date

Chapter Three

A HOME CAREGIVER FOR ME?

" 'Mrs. Roebuck,' age 72, was losing weight and had memory problems that seemed to be worsening. She was getting lost in her own neighborhood; recently she had been unable to find her way home and wandered for several hours.

Lee, Mrs. Roebuck's daughter, found Clara through a newspaper advertisement. Clara made meals, tidied the house and did some shopping. When Lee's mother was not having a good day, Clara would insist on staying overnight to care for her.

Mrs. Roebuck now lives in a retirement complex, with 24-hour staff on duty. She no longer recognizes Clara when she comes to visit. But, thanks to her daughter and this dedicated home caregiver, Mrs. Roebuck was able to live one extra year in her own home."

— Bruce Thomas, Geriatric Care Manager

THE STORY ABOVE ILLUSTRATES WHAT WE ALL TRY HARD NOT to think about when it comes to aging loved ones. Is it time to put Mother in a nursing home? Should she move in with us? Who pays for long term care? Confronting questions like these is certainly one of life's most difficult dilemmas.

Sooner or later, this crisis of decision-making will confront most families. When it does, you will wish to consider all your options. And, you would be well-advised to seek professional advice and consultation.

Mrs. Roebuck, with her confusion and other symptoms, was in the early stages of Alzheimer's disease. (About 10 percent of persons over the age of 65 will be afflicted by a similar or related condition.) While she did not require medical treatment, she did need supervision and assistance. Although a steady decline in her condition could be expected, her health did not vary too much day-to-day. She met nearly all of the criteria for hiring a home caregiver.

Other elders could benefit from the services of a home caregiver because of a health condition that limits their ability to perform routine tasks. People with back or spine problems, arthritis, and heart and stroke conditions in particular, may need help with getting around, with housework and with meal preparation.

Other physical limitations include difficulty lifting heavy objects, trouble climbing stairs, and problems with vision or hearing. In general, people who cannot get around easily, or who need help getting into or out of a tub or a bed are likely to need in-home assistance.

CHECKLIST FOR HIRING A HOME CAREGIVER
Help Needed with Routine Tasks
- Dressing/undressing
- Keeping clean and presentable
- Toileting
- Housework

Help Needed with Meals
- Cooking
- Special diets
- Need for adequate liquids
- Help with feeding

Help Needed with Medications
- Taking medications as prescribed

Help Needed with Household Affairs
- Records management
- Transportation
- Escort to appointments
- Banking

Help Needed by Caregivers
- Caregiver is ill
- Caregiver at work
- Caregiver needs respite

Special Concerns
- Confusion and disorientation
- Mental health issues

You can be as successful as Lee in finding and keeping a home caregiver. But first, you should obtain professional recommendations. This will help alleviate some of the uncertainty of decision-making, and will give you the peace of mind of knowing that you have chosen a workable plan. Start by seeing your doctor. Then, consult with a geriatric care manager.

Of course professional services can be expensive. While a doctor's fee is often covered by Medicare, there are few reimbursement systems in place for care management. One option for families on a budget is to check with the local Area Agency on Aging. Oftentimes, these federally and state funded agencies can send out a case worker to do an initial in-home assessment at no charge.

Is a Medical Check-up Needed?

A complete and thorough medical examination is always called for when an elder begins to struggle with once simple tasks. Good doctors will never say "What can you expect at her age?" They will take the time to get to the bottom of the difficulty, and suggest ways to remedy it.

You may wish to schedule a consultation with a physician specializing in geriatric medicine. "Geriatric specialists" can play an important role in assessing the feasibility of home care for the very old, or those with complex chronic health problems. They can provide the results of their assessment to the family doctor, who can then continue to provide care for the elder patient.

It's not too hard to find a doctor, particularly an internist, psychiatrist or family practitioner, who is board certified in treating the needs and problems of older people. To become board certified in geriatrics, a doctor has met rigorous professional standards, has completed a residency in geriatrics and has successfully completed examinations.

Three good ways to locate a geriatric specialist: call a college of medicine in your area; call your county medical society; or call the American Geriatrics Society in New York City at (212) 308-1414.

Lee had taken her mother to a medical clinic specializing in memory disorders for a complete mental and physical evaluation. She also had her mother evaluated by a *geriatric care manager* to discuss the workability of home care.

What Is a "Geriatric Care Manager"?

Some gerontologists, social workers, and nurses are now providing a service called "care management." These professionals evaluate an elder's needs, discuss options, and link families with services. The emphasis is on a personalized approach and ongoing contact with the elder and family by phone, letter and/or personal visits.

Care managers determine the right "mix" of services. (You won't be told to hire a nurse when a home caregiver would do, for instance.) Generally during the first few visits, the care manager helps identify needs and discusses the pros and cons of each option for care. Then, he or she will assist you in arranging for services to begin.

The care manager also will stay in touch over several months, if you like, to make sure that services are in place, well managed, and meet needs.

What Do Care Managers Do?

Care managers provide a complete range of services: assessment for community-based or institutional placement, referral and coordination of services, assistance with forms and applications, hiring and monitoring of staff and ongoing supervision. Their services can be of vital importance when it comes to implementing home care. The steps listed below are typical of the process that a care manager will go through in planning for in-home care.

Assessment

Work begins with an in-depth evaluation to assess the elder's ability to function around the house. The goal is to understand the degree of difficulty the elder has in managing ordinary activities. A simple Scale of Abilities that a care manager might use as a part of an assessment can be found at the end of this chapter.

Care Planning

After assessing the elder's situation at home, along with her social and economic status, the care manager writes out a plan of care, which could include the hiring of a home helper, along with other services that will help the elder manage independently. The plan of care spells out the type, level and frequency of services. This plan should always include the expectations and choices of the elder and family.

Coordination of Care

If the elder's problems are complex and changing, a variety of services may be needed. In cases like these, the care manager can perform much like an orchestra conductor, blending and directing harmonious arrangements of service over time.

Monitoring of Services

After the home caregiver has started her job, the care manager can, if you like, keep in touch to monitor the quality of care provided to the elder. He or she can ensure that home care workers appear as scheduled, and perform their tasks skillfully and honestly. Particularly in instances where the elder lives miles away from her family, it is important to have a permanent contact with a local professional who can assist in the ongoing monitoring of services.

Reassessment

Because the elder's needs change over time, her condition will need to be periodically re-evaluated. For example, once an elder is determined to be a good candidate for home care, subsequent assessments could be conducted at six month or yearly intervals. Of course, any noticeable change in an elder's condition always calls for reassessment.

How Do I Find a Geriatric Care Manager?

In larger cities, care managers may be located by simply checking the yellow pages of the local phone directory. Otherwise, contact hospitals, professional associations, information and referral services, and in some areas, Area Agencies on Aging. Ask your hospital's discharge planner for referrals. You might also contact state departments of aging, family service agencies or a national association of professionals. Check Appendix G for information on how to get in touch with a care manager in your area.

While there is some reassurance in knowing that a care manager works for a long-established and reputable agency, working with a private practitioner represents an attractive alternative. Care managers working for themselves (self-employed) can be every bit as qualified as agency workers and often charge lower fees.

Because this is a new and developing field, there are as yet no widely-recognized standards for licensure, certification, accreditation and other forms of quality assurance. This holds true for care managers working for themselves, working in small private businesses or in larger companies. When choosing a care manager, carefully consider background, experience, and references. Work with an individual who holds a master's degree in social work, nursing, gerontology, psychology or counseling, who has at least three years of experience and who is licensed in his or her particular field.

If you are dealing with a private practitioner rather than an agency-affiliated care manager, even greater care is needed to select the most reputable professional. Check with the Better Business Bureau and, if money will be handled, run a credit check and ask if the care manager is bonded. (Also see "Questions to Ask When Hiring a Private Care Manager" on page 33).

What Does Care Management Cost?

Rates range from $50 an hour and up, and are sometimes negotiable between the care manager, elder and family. Charges may be hourly, a flat annual rate, a per service fee or, occasionally with agencies, a sliding charge adjusted according to your ability to pay. Medicare and most private insurances do not reimburse for geriatric care management. This means that payment will mostly come out of your income or assets.

You might get by with just a single in-home visit and initial assessment. As assessments usually require several hours of interviewing and the completion of a written report, it may cost in the neighborhood of two to three hundred dollars. In many cases, once the initial assessment has been completed, families can handle the on-going coordination and monitoring of care themselves.

You may locate another source of professionals able to provide a geriatric assessment by calling your Area Agency on Aging. Some of these agencies can do an assessment for you with their own staff, while others will refer you to an agency which will do so. In either case, this route can offer a less expensive alternative. Note: Some long-term care insurance policies will pay for or provide a geriatric assessment. As a final low-cost alternative, it's important to realize that home health agencies can provide an assessment for you. There is normally no charge if you become a patient.

While fees may seem high, you can actually save money by working through a care manager. He or she can reduce overuse of services and inappropriate placement in long term care facilities. Matching services to an elder's needs helps contain costs. Ongoing monitoring can prevent costly crises and unnecessary hospitalizations.

When a Home Caregiver Is Not a Good Idea

The home caregiver option should be pursued only if such an arrangement has a reasonably good chance of working out. In situations where safety and security would be compromised, it's *never* a good idea.

It is difficult to describe cases in which the home care option is inappropriate because each situation is unique. Here are some indicators, however, that may signal that a family may have difficulty in providing on-going care that is sufficient for the elder's well-being. In such cases, relocation to a more supportive setting may be the best option — both for the safety of the elder and the peace of mind of family members.

- *24-hour care and supervision needed.* Most families, even with the backup of two or more helpers, cannot successfully provide constant, round-the-clock care. This kind of day and night protective supervision is often needed to keep the severely confused person from hazards and dangers in the home environment.
- *Movement requires two helpers.* With a bedridden person, the danger of falls, muscle strain, and injury

is great — for both elder and helper. Untrained persons should not attempt to provide care to an immobile elder who is confined to bed.

- *Deteriorating health.* The need for relocation may be precipitated by the progressive decline associated with diseases like Alzheimer's, or may involve a crisis, such as a fall or stroke. Eventually, for some of us, the time does come when halfway measures are no longer enough. Sadly, with Alzheimer's cases, nursing home placement is usually a question of "when" rather than "if."

- *Changes in family status.* In many cases, the managerial services provided by family members are vital to the success of a program of self-directed eldercare. For a variety of reasons, family members may become incapacitated when it comes to providing practical and emotional support to elders.

The "Scale of Abilities" that follows may also help you form an initial impression of the suitability of a home caregiver in your particular situation

A SCALE OF ABILITIES

Rank 1: Independent
   Requires no help from another person
   Safety not at risk

Rank 2: Needs Verbal Assistance
   Reminding/guidance required
   Hands-on help not needed

Rank 3: Needs Minimal Assistance
   Needs some direct hands-on care

Rank 4: Needs Significant Assistance
   Needs a great deal of help from another person

Rank 5: Needs Total Assistance
  Requires total care
  Totally dependent upon another person

Rank 6: Needs Medical Services
  Respiratory suctioning
  Tube feedings
  Ostomy/catheter care; other care
  Wound care

If we were to apply the Scale of Abilities to Mrs. Roebuck's case related at the beginning of this chapter, here's how it might look:

TASK	RANK	HELP NEEDED
Housework	4	Needs significant help
Laundry	4	Need significant help
Shopping and errands	5	Cannot perform without assistance
Meal prep. and clearing	4	Needs significant help
Mobility inside	1	Independent
Bathing and grooming	4	Needs significant help
Elimination	2	Needs verbal assistance
Eating	1	Independent

These rankings make Mrs. Roebuck's need for help in housework and bathing obvious; otherwise she appears to be someone who could manage safely at home with minimal assistance. She is a good candidate for a home helper arrangement. Total assistance is needed in only one area: transportation.

On the other hand, if Mrs. Roebuck was assessed with mostly 5's (requires total care) or 6's (needs medical services) she would not be an appropriate candidate for home care. Other arrangements would then need to be considered: having the elder live with someone else, or having someone live with her; or, relocating her to one of the many community-based residential alternatives available for older people (board and care homes, continuing care retirement community or a long-term care institution).

* * * * * *

This chapter has introduced you to the complexities of assessing for home care. To make an informed decision about relocation versus in-home services, it's necessary to assess a number of factors:

- The elder's current health status.
- The economic resources available.
- With help, can the elder can manage her environment despite age-related impairments?
- The mental status of the elder. Is she forgetful? Can she safely remain in her own home?
- Finally, we need to understand her extended network of family, friends and community support. Even the most dedicated home helper can't meet all an elder's needs without family assistance.

By taking the time and effort to explore all the available options with the assistance of a professional geriatric care manager, most families will be able to develop a good plan for in-home care. The process is never easy, but, more often than not, careful evaluation and planning will make it possible for the older person to continue to manage at home.

QUESTIONS TO ASK A CARE MANAGER

1. How much experience do you have in care management?

2. Do you have a professional license (social worker, nurse, counselor, etc.)?

3. Can you provide references (such as hospitals or senior centers)?

4. Do you carry professional liability insurance? Are you bonded?

5. How often can I expect reports? Written or phoned?

6. What are your fees and what do they include (e.g., initial assessment, care plan, coordination)?

7. Do you provide a written contract specifying fees/services?

8. What is your caseload? (20-30 clients is about average)

RECRUITING YOUR HELPER

"My husband has high blood pressure, sugar, and is recovering from two heart attacks. He can't stay by himself, although he eats well and sleeps good. I've got to get out for a couple of hours. We've been married sixty-three years, but I think I still have a little life left to live. The agency I called charges $11.85 per hour; after scrimping and scraping all our lives, we can't afford that. Wouldn't someone want to watch him and earn a few dollars?"

— Mrs. Reed, age 82, homemaker

IT IS NEVER EASY TO FIND THE IDEAL HOME HELPER. THERE ARE good, honest, and reliable people out there, but you've got to seek them out — they rarely appear at your doorstep.

Recruitment can be done effectively in only one way: "sweat equity." When recruitment is done in a thorough and methodical way, as outlined in this chapter, the end result is likely to be a match that's comfortable for everyone. For those who take shortcuts and the "easy chair" approach, disappointment is almost certain.

For some people, employment as a home caregiver represents a convenient way to temporarily make ends meet. These workers tend to "drift" into homecare and quit their jobs just as soon as something better comes along. Indeed, one of the major problems in home care is the high employee turnover rate.

Others have more of a lasting commitment. In addition to the advantages of this type of work — flexibility, for instance — they really like working with older adults. They can handle the more mundane and demanding aspects of the job because they realize they are providing indispensable assistance. They have a strong preference for an occupation that allows them to care for another person. This is the kind of home caregiver you want to find.

The "Right" Person for the Job
Certain character and personality traits define the ideal home caregiver. They may be thought of as the "5 Cs":

- *Caring.* It is essential that the home caregiver genuinely respect, like, and appreciate the special qualities of older people. Empathy and sympathy are part of this — not pity. Additionally, she must be the kind of person who finds helping others personally rewarding. Look for the home caregiver who expresses sentiments like the following: "I feel wanted and needed when working with older people." "I like to help older people; I might need help someday when I'm older." "I feel that I can improve how an older person lives."

- *Conscientious.* When a home caregiver is hired she is agreeing to take on awesome responsibility, for the well-being of another person is in her hands. The most basic requirement is that she be someone you can count on. In other words, 98% of the time, she will come to work when scheduled, be on time and give advance notice when unable to work. And because of the isolated nature of the home environment, an in-home caregiver must be honest. You must feel comfortable in entrusting her with access to an elder's home and possessions.

- *Competent*. The home caregiver should have the capacity to provide personal care in a tolerant and matter of fact way. She should be able to handle stressful situations without becoming upset. She must also make good judgments. For instance, in an emergency situation the home caregiver must be able to decide whether to call the doctor, call 911 or go to the emergency room.

- *Compassionate*. In addition to being caring, conscientious and competent, it helps immensely if the caregiver is patient, sensitive, a listener, gentle and compassionate. Older people don't hurry so easily, so patience is a must when working with them. After a lifetime of practice, elders tend to be very discerning when it comes to genuineness and warmth that are demonstrated through actions as well as words.

- *Considerate*. The best caregiver adapts to an elder's lifestyle without being rigid in her ideas about how things should be done. In other words, she must be able to follow instructions while maintaining a pleasant attitude. It's marvelous if, occasionally, the caregiver will adjust her hours to provide evening, weekend and holiday care.

Research has pinpointed which personality traits are most helpful in caregiving relationships. The "5 Cs" are some of the most important.

Where Should You Look?

You can shorten the recruiting process by concentrating on those pools of potential employees that are the most likely to yield results. The idea is to target those persons suited by experience and life circumstance to helping elders. Professional recruiters have had success with students and young, middle age, or older women.

Middle-aged and older women in particular are the focus of most recruitment efforts because of their experience in nurturing and homemaking roles. Women represent the bulk of the long-term care workforce. Of course, there are exceptions to this rule. Men, for instance, can and do provide excellent care to older people. Male care recipients in particular, sometimes prefer being tended to by another man.

Here are some ideas on promising labor pools.

Students and Young Adults

Many high school or college students are looking for part-time jobs to cover expenses. Although they may lack experience, they often make good caregivers. This kind of work is often ideally suited to college students' schedules. Sometimes students in nursing, rehabilitation, physical therapy and related fields are looking for practical experience.

Women with Young Children

Increasingly, both parents work; but there are still many parents at home with young children. Women whose young children are in school, or can be left in childcare settings, often bring a good deal of understanding and skill to home helper work. They are good candidates for part-time jobs.

Mature Women

Mature women often make wonderful home helpers because, after raising their own families, they have a real feel for caretaking.

Some mature women fall into the category of "displaced homemakers." They have "lost their jobs" through widowhood, separation or divorce. Matching an elder with a displaced homemaker sometimes meets the needs of both sets of people.

A study conducted by the Commonwealth Fund of New York indicated that there may be up to 1.9 million older people who are ready and willing to work. When asked what jobs they would be willing to take, over 60% said they would like to provide services to older people in their own homes. Other research has shown that mature workers are more likely to stay on the job as compared to younger workers.

Retirees

Retirees seek employment because they need part-time work to supplement their income, or because they wish to help others, or both. Of course, older workers must have the level of fitness needed to assist with personal care services and household tasks. Older workers tend to be the most reliable of all workers. And, sometimes "older people know better how to care for older people."

It's important to note that, for those who are retired but continue to work, earnings may affect Social Security benefits. Annual earnings limits apply to everyone who gets Social Security checks except those who are 70 years of age or older.

In general, your home caregiver will receive all the Social Security benefits due her if her wages do not exceed the following 1995 limits:

- For people under the age of 65, the limit is $8,160.
- For people age 65 through 69, the limit is $11,280.

Above these limits, benefits are reduced $1.00 for every $2.00 earned over the limit. Call the SSA for current rates.

Recent Immigrants

The large pool of recent immigrants to the United States is an excellent source of home care assistance. Some immigrants are not fully documented, of course, so it is important to avoid the potential legal and tax issues related to hiring an illegal alien (knowingly or unknowingly). Precautions necessary to prevent problems with immigration officials and the IRS will be reviewed in Chapter 10.

Ethnic Populations

The majority of home caregiver jobs are filled by women who are African-American, Hispanic, or members of other ethnic groups. It is worth noting that social and cultural beliefs that reinforce such values as extended families, respect for older persons, and in-home care are often stronger among women of non-Anglo cultures.

Recruitment can begin at public agencies, at training programs and schools, or at organizations which promote employment opportunities for members of various cultural and ethnic groups.

What Basic Qualifications Should You Require?

Employees gravitate toward home caregiver work for different reasons; one is that, somewhere along the line, they've encountered barriers to employment. These range from being considered too young or too old, or being under-experienced or over-experienced. Other major barriers are not speaking or reading English and/or being on public assistance.

Avoid the trap of unrealistic expectations. Good judgment, honesty, and dependability can be found in those who have never graduated from high school. And, don't rule out people who have previously been receiving public assistance or unemployment benefits. Agencies have demonstrated that workers who have no work history at all can be successfully trained in home care skills.

Here are some basic requirements:
- Speaks language of elder
- Reads simple instructions
- 18 years of age (see page 154 for exceptions)
- Good physical and mental health
- Good moral character
- Possesses a Social Security card (excludes undocumented aliens from employment)

Should You Use an Employment Registry?

In general, employment registries and referral pools provide a base to help locate in-home help. Some registries are simple listings of names; others provide screening, billing services and background checks. (In either case, the *user* of the service most often retains all the rights, responsibilities, and liabilities that go along with the employer role.) When calling an employment registry, it is important to inquire about screening processes and training requirements, as well as about any fees charged.

The advantage of using an employment pool or registry is quick access to a list of potential applicants. When you need a home caregiver, you can contact the service, which will provide you with a list of people looking for work. You still have the full right to select or pass over the applicants as you choose, and you can usually negotiate the salary (if it has not been pre-set) on a case-by-case basis. These systems do provide a convenient way for workers and employers to link up with one another.

Should You Use an Employment Agency?

Commercial employment agencies, for a fee, recruit, screen and test potential employees. Sometimes the placement fee is charged to the worker; sometimes to the employer. The exact nature of the arrangement will probably be specified in a contract or business agreement.

Employment agencies may or may not be licensed by the state in which they do business. A license does offer a certain peace of mind. For one thing, all state-licensed agencies must carry a bond. A license also helps ensure that the agency honors guarantees connected with fees charged. If an agency misrepresents any part of a placement fee, it jeopardizes its state license.

Employment agencies screen and test potential employees drawn from a wide field of candidates. They relieve you of much of the time and effort involved in recruiting a home helper. But, let the buyer beware. Check out the agency's reputation with the Better Business Bureau, and ask to see references from past or current clients.

What If You Want To Recruit on Your Own?

Recruitment is the first step for those who have decided to undertake consumer-directed home care. This merely involves getting the notice of your job opening out to as many likely candidates as you can. You can use the strategy that most agencies use (placing an advertisement in the newspaper), or you can save money and find your helper the old-fashioned way, namely "through the grapevine." Both methods will yield good results.

If you decide to try recruiting on your own, the four basic strategies available to you include:
- Advertising in newspapers
- Posting flyers
- Recruiting by telephone
- Word of mouth

Advertising in Newspapers

Do not assume that the fastest and easiest way to find a caregiver is to place an ad in your local newspaper. Be aware that, when using this technique, you will be competing with the many home care agencies that rely mainly upon ads as their sole recruitment tactic. Newspaper ads tend to generate many responses very quickly, but 90 percent of these respondents may be unsuitable. And many of the individuals you are targeting in your recruitment efforts, including senior citizens, often don't read help-wanted ads.

Don't rule out newspaper ads entirely, however. The classified ad department in most papers will help you write an ad, but if you write your own — one that really attracts callers — you may get better results. The following suggestions will help you make the most of your ad:

- *Make your job sound appealing.* Give a feeling of what kind of family you are. (Warm, caring people respond to ads that sound caring.) Highlight the attractive features of the position (extra income, flexible hours).

- *Include any perks you may be offering* (paid vacations, meals, transportation, no heavy housework required).

- *Consider an answering service.* Don't give too much information. Rather than listing your home phone number, consider hiring an answering service which will assign a number for your use. This eliminates some of the risk of giving out your home or office number.

- *Do not list your address.* This will prevent applicants from showing up on your doorstep.

- *Consider renting a post office box.* This way you avoid having to publish your name or phone number in the advertisement. If you require that applicants respond to a post office box, you limit the volume of response.

- *Never list your last name!*

- *State the hours you can be reached.* You may wish to be contacted after work hours if you are employed, but you'll have a better response if you make yourself available for a wider range of hours.

- *Get advice from the newspaper staff.* Ask the newspaper's ad representative to help you place your ad in the best section. He or she can also provide good suggestions about headline size, and the use of graphics, borders and large or bold type.

And, as mentioned previously, the ad sales representative can help you with writing and re-writing your "help-wanted" ad. Let this advertising expert help you fit the maximum amount of information into a minimal cost-per-line space. Use abbreviations when possible (for example, using PO instead of post office means you pay for one word instead of two.)

Consider placing the ad in the Part-time, Health Care, Household, or Domestic Help Wanted section. Sundays and Wednesdays are good days to run ads. A week-long advertisement will generate a good sized list of applicants from which to choose. Place the ad in city newspapers; college, neighborhood and community newspapers and/or newspapers that target specific ethnic groups.

Sample Ads

At a minimum, your ad should include the name of the position, hours needed, a brief description of duties, and contact information. You should also mention preferences such as non-smoker, male/female, the wage you are offering and any needed experience or qualifications.

Here are some examples that you can modify to suit your own needs and preferences:

HOME HELPER WANTED: Dependable person to provide personal care and grocery shopping for older adult, 7-10 am M-F. $4.25/hour. Call Jim at (phone number).

EXCELLENT FOR STUDENT: Aide for retired older couple. Shopping, housework and personal care. 6-10 a.m. M-W-F. $___hr. phone no.___ Ref. req., non-smoker.

IN-HOME AIDE: Good location, near bus route; Housekeeping and some personal care for older man who uses wheelchair. Salary for 5 days/wk., 6 hrs. a day available for right person. No experience needed. Respond in writing to PO Box ____.

SPECIAL CAREGIVER for my confused, 89 year old mother. Part-time, must be willing to cook and provide some transportation. $150/wk. Call Abby (phone number).

NOTE: Don't forget to check the "situations wanted" column in the classified advertisement section of the newspaper. You may find that just the person you are looking for is busy looking for you!

Recruiting through Posted Flyers

Neatly type your flyer, or print it in bold lettering on eye-catching paper. Place the flyer at eye level so that it is easier to see. Make sure that the lettering, especially the heading, is visible from a distance. Use a staple gun when permitted, one staple in each corner of the flyer. (Tacks stand a good chance of being borrowed by the next person who forgot to bring their own.)

Post your flyer on bulletin boards in the following places.
- Houses of worship
- College dormitories
- Libraries
- Supermarkets

- YMCA/YWCA
- Vocational rehabilitation agencies
- Hospitals
- Senior centers
- Mobile home parks
- Apartment complexes
- Retirement communities
- Health care clinics
- Cultural centers

NOTE: A sample flyer/job announcement can be found at the end of this chapter.

Recruiting by Telephone

A great deal of ground may be covered by using your telephone for some targeted recruitment. A few well-placed calls may net you several good candidates to interview.

Training programs. Many vocational and trade schools have placement offices. Call to see if they have graduates that you can interview.

Employment, training and referral services. State employment offices may offer free public employment services, including listings for household employment. Displaced homemaker services and private industry councils often place youth, women and older workers.

Local chapters of national health associations. Cancer, heart, or lung disease; diabetes; and Parkinson's and Alzheimer's disease are among the conditions for which national organizations have local chapters. Some maintain listings of those seeking employment.

Independent living centers. "ILCs" are community centers that serve the needs of disabled persons of all ages. If you live in an area that is served by an ILC, try obtaining the names and phone numbers of those who may have listed their names as available as personal care attendants. Be sure to spell out any special physical requirements for care of your elder (e.g., lifting).

Senior employment programs. National employment services such as the Senior Community Service Employment Program through AARP, train and place older workers. Other programs include "Senior Companion," the Job Training and Partnership Act, and Title V senior employment programs. Call your local Area Agency on Aging for information.

High schools. Call in an announcement to the guidance or career development center of local high schools. Some schools have employment centers housed in their library.

Colleges. Most colleges have a "job book" in which you may post your job opening. In most instances all you have to do is call the school's information office to get the name of the right department on campus, and then give them the information over the phone. Don't overlook college "life-long learning" departments that attract mature students.

Information and referral systems. "I&Rs "do not specialize in home care per se; they are an all-purpose community reference point. They may be able to refer you, however, to agencies that can send job-seekers your way. Check the phone book under such listings as "Information and Referral Service," "Senior Citizen's Services," "Community Service," "Action Lines," "Hot Line," "CONTACT," "HELP," or ask your local telephone information operator for assistance.

Community services. Look in the telephone directory under "community services." Look for private, government or church-related programs that serve minorities and new immigrants. These organizations include cultural community centers and healthcare clinics. Call to ask if you can mail in a job announcement.

Recruiting by Word of Mouth

A well-developed "informal network" exists in the field of home care, just as it does in the corporate world and other parts of our society. Recruitment experts swear by the word of mouth approach as the single most effective strategy to discover the ideal home caregiver. Perhaps the best jobs and the best workers are never written up in advertisements at all, but are merely referred from friend to friend, family to family. Let the grapevine work for you! Here are some ideas to get you started:

Relatives, friends and co-workers. If you do a little digging, you will find that many people know of good home caregivers. Ask your friends to keep their eyes and ears open for anyone who may be looking for a job.

Personal recommendations. Personal recommendations are often the best because you'll get a feel for the worker's personal habits. Check with families that have previously employed in-home help.

Your doctor. In addition to the doctor, often the doctor's nurse, or other staff who work with patients, can help direct you to good in-home workers.

Local clergy. Some local churches and synagogues provide direct home care services to their members, or provide registry services for those looking for work.

Professionals at work. If you are employed, or are a company retiree, check with your employee benefits or human resources manager.

Other home helpers. Presently employed home caregivers can often recommend good candidates. More job seekers find out about jobs through friends than through newspaper ads or other sources.

Support groups. Attending a self-help support group is one of the best ways to gain inside information on services and service providers, including home caregivers.

* * * * * *

As the demand grows for basic in-home services, so will the competition in recruitment of good home caregivers. Anyone seeking to place their hat in the recruitment ring must contend with competition from home care agencies large and small.

To successfully beat businesses at their own game, you've got to know where helpers are likely to be found and how to make contact with them. You've got to hone your recruitment message so that it communicates simply and effectively, focusing on the practical benefits of your job opening. You can compete more effectively if you are able to offer some of the benefits employees have come to expect when they work for larger organizations: Worker's Compensation and health care insurance, retirement contributions, paid vacation time, perhaps even housing and meals.

One of the best ways to sharpen your efforts is to understand the position and interests of those individuals who are likely to be looking for in-home employment. The more you can tailor your job in a way that maximizes tangible benefits to them, the better your chances of winning the recruitment game.

With persistence and luck, there's a good chance of finding someone within one to two weeks. A more complicated situation, fewer hours, lower pay and fewer benefits will all make the search more difficult.

Recruitment is not a process for folks who are easily discouraged. To be successful, you'll have to cultivate every possible connection: from the print media, to the telephone, to the "grapevine." You'll be rewarded by achieving the goal you are pursuing: making contact with a conscientious, competent and considerate job applicant, and especially someone who truly cares.

(SAMPLE FLYER)

Please Post

IN-HOME HELPER WANTED

Our family is looking for a warm, caring person
to help our elderly mother in her own home.

Job Description:
- Part-time, MWF, 9:00 - 1:00
- Personal care, light housekeeping
- Occasional weekends

Salary: $120 per week

Benefits: Lunches, Car allowance

Job Requirements:
- Non-smoker
- Trustworthy
- Position begins October 1st
- Clean driving record

Qualifications:
- Experienced with elders
- Excellent references
- No criminal or abuse record

If interested, please call Mrs. Vinsonhaler
after 6:00 p.m. at 555-1234

---

*NOTE: To make your phone number convenient to those who are
interested but are without paper or pencil, consider using "tear tabs"at the
bottom of your flyer that give the name of the position and your phone
number (for example: "In-Home Helper: 555-1234").*

Chapter Five

_____

SELECTING YOUR CAREGIVER

"I dust, clean the kitchen and his bathroom, mop his floors, do his laundry and change his bed. I open and set drinks for him in the refrigerator and meals and snacks so that he can feed himself without burning himself or spilling too much. If I didn't look after him this way, he couldn't live on his own."

— Geneva Black, Home Helper for Mr. Jones, age 97

INTERVIEWING POTENTIAL HOME CAREGIVERS CAN OFTEN feel like a huge and confusing task. You can simplify the process by dividing it into smaller steps. This will allow you more time to think over and talk over the information that you gather from applicants. Every family has different needs, but by following a four-step approach you can select the home caregiver that best suits you.

Step One   Telephone Screening

Step Two   Conducting the Interview

Step Three   Checking References

Step Four   Making the Job Offer

Telephone Screening

Those who call to inquire about the job should be thoroughly "screened" before a face-to-face interview is scheduled. This means that you will separate those whom cannot meet your needs from those whom you will interview personally. This saves time for both you and the caller, and lays the groundwork for selecting the ideal home helper. *Initial telephone screening is one of the most important steps in selecting your home caregiver!*

Here are some tips for conducting telephone screenings:

Answer the telephone in a friendly manner. Attempt to paint a realistic picture of the job, so that the caller has few misconceptions. Describe the salary, duties, days & hours needed, and the general location of the home (not the address!).

This step weeds out those who want a higher salary and those who aren't available at the time that you need them. You might also want to screen out callers who live outside comfortable reach of public transportation (depending on the availability and reliability of your local transportation system.) This reduces the likelihood of transportation problems. For those who respond favorably, continue the screening process. Ask quick questions to gather basic facts. Take down the information in writing. Use copies of the "Telephone Screening Worksheet" on the following page to collect and organize information.

Next, ask about school-work, past employment and any special training. (If work record does not account for years between high school and present, find out how the caller has been spending her time.) Look for at least one year of experience related to personal care.

Ask a few open-ended questions (questions that cannot be answered by a simple " yes" or "no"). For example, you might ask about any previous jobs or experience that involved caregiving. Ask something like "What were the things you liked best about working with older people?"

TELEPHONE SCREENING WORKSHEET

Date _____

Caller's name_____

Address_____

_____

Home phone number_____ Age_____

Are you currently working?_____

Where have you worked before?_____

_____

_____

Can you provide verifiable work references?_____

Do you have experience as a home helper?_____

_____

_____

Do you have a Social Security number?_____

Do you have a driver's license?_____

How long have you lived in this area?_____

Open-ended questions_____

_____

_____

_____

Notes_____

_____

_____

Listen closely to the style and timing of her responses. Does she understand your questions? Does she answer questions easily? Or, is she guarded and hesitant?

If you are still interested, go on to describe the position in detail. Be specific, listing duties such as bathing, dressing, cooking, cleaning, and whatever else is required. Stress that the job is much more than household maintenance, involving personal care of an older person. Ask how the caller feels about working with frail elders. This kind of discussion will help you gauge the applicant's overall comfort level with personal care issues.

The final step of telephone screening is to conclude the telephone contact:
Thank the caller for responding, and for her interest in the job — even if she is obviously unsuitable. (You may want to file certain names and address; they may come in handy in the future.) Tell each caller that you're still screening job-seekers over the phone, and when you have finished with this process, IF YOU ARE INTERESTED, you will get back in touch:

"I appreciate your interest in this position, Mrs. Smith. I'm still taking calls about the job. **If I'm interested***, I'll be calling you in a few days to schedule an interview. If you don't hear from me, you'll know I won't be inviting you to interview. Thanks very much for calling."*

Although problems stemming from telephone screenings are unlikely, you must be on the alert when dealing with strangers. Always withhold information on your name and address. Don't answer calls in the middle of the night, (unless you're the only coverage for your elder). You may want to unplug your phone after bedtime hours. If any caller doesn't respond when you answer, hang up. If any caller makes you feel uneasy, just use the, "If you don't hear from me..." statement above.

After inquiries about the job have subsided, look through your Telephone Screening Worksheets, and rank them according to your notes and personal impressions. Compare the callers both with each other and with your needs.

Through this initial screening process, you should be able to narrow your choices. To increase your chances of successfully choosing a home caregiver, it is important to set up formal interviews with no fewer than three candidates. Call each of these job candidates back and schedule the interview:

• Arrange to meet with the job candidates at a public location, a restaurant for example. The idea is to choose some neutral spot other than your home.

• Ask each candidate to bring identification, Social Security card, summary of employment history, proof of address (i.e., rent bill) to the interview, along with job and personal reference contact information. If driving will be a part of the job, you may wish to ask the candidate to furnish proof of a clear driving record (she can obtain a form from the motor vehicle department).

• Ask candidates to please call if they change their minds or if they are otherwise unable to keep the appointment.

Conducting the Interview

If at all possible, take another person (friend, family member, neighbor or advisor) with you to the interview. This person's task is simply to observe the entire exchange as perceptively as possible. While you are busy reading the job application and filling out the interview questionnaire, he or she can focus on how the job applicant conducts herself. In this way, the second interviewer will gain valuable first impressions on the potential home helper's appearance, manner and tone of voice. Two heads really are better than one, and it helps to have a second opinion.

Give yourself forty-five to sixty minutes per interview. If you use the application form beginning on page 57, add another fifteen to thirty minutes.

When the job applicant arrives, set her at ease by offering her a beverage or use of the rest room. Next, have her fill out the employment application. The form will provide you with summary information about both her experience and background.

Begin the formal interview process by checking the application for completeness. Go over it carefully "point by point" with the job seeker, commenting on any answers that seem vague, unusual or for which you would like further information.

After reviewing and discussing the application, you are ready to begin asking very specific questions. The questions listed on the interview questionnaire included in this chapter have been "field tested" and proven effective for eliciting the most telling and relevant information. You will be writing down your notes on the form throughout this guided interview. The idea is to gain as much revealing and relevant information from the candidate as you can.

Secrets of a Successful Interview
• Here is a quick checklist of how to conduct an efficient and successful interview:
• Prior to interviewing, review all your questions.
• Start the interview on time.
• Stay on track so that you can gather the maximum amount of information in the time allotted.
• Listen more and talk less. The bulk of interview time should be devoted to listening.
• Never make a job offer on the spot; keep your options open.
• Tell job seekers that you will check all references before making a job offer.

• Take time immediately after the interview to fill out the "First Impressions Worksheet" found later in this chapter.

• Discuss your impressions with the other observer present at the interview. Compare notes. Take all comments and viewpoints into consideration. Consider the effects upon the elder of hiring a certain person.

• Trust your first impressions and personal reactions.

• Don't be surprised if the job-seeker also "interviews" you — the relationship between a home helper and family is very special. You both need to feel comfortable about your partnership.

Concluding the Interview

If you feel the candidate might suit your needs, let her know that you are definitely interested and that you will get back to her. Make sure you give her a time frame of when you'll get back. This should be no longer than one to five days.

Should You Require an Employment Application?

All job seekers should complete an application in your presence, immediately before the interview. This will help you check for neatness, English-language skills and general educational level. It will also record information in a systematic way, and serve as a signed release form for eventually conducting background checks.

Another reason that the combined application/interview approach is so effective is that it allows you to double check the information. For example, you can probe for further information on any written response that seems questionable to you, or for which you would like more details.

The sample "Employment Application" form on the following pages may be useful if you wish to follow this suggested approach to selecting your caregiver. You may also find pre-printed forms in a local stationery store.

EMPLOYMENT APPLICATION

Name_____
      first   middle   last   (maiden)

Social Security #_____ Phone #_____

Address_____

City/State/Zip_____

How long have you lived in this area?_____

How will you get to and from work?_____

Driver's License #_____ Car license #_____

Car make & year *(if driving will be required)*_____

Education

High School_____Date Graduated_____

College_____Dates Attended_____

Degree_____Major field_____

Other Training or Courses_____

Caregiving Experience (list most recent employer first)

•Employer_____
    Date: From_____To_____
    Employer Phone #_____Position_____
    Reason for Leaving_____
_____
_____

• Employer_____

    Date: From_____To_____

    Employer Phone#_____Position_____

    Reason for Leaving_____

_____

_____

• Employer_____

    Date: From_____To_____

    Employer Phone#_____Position_____

    Reason for Leaving_____

_____

_____

What days and hours are you available?_____

Are you available for extra hours?_____

Why do you want to be a home caregiver?_____

_____

Have you ever been charged any violations including traffic?_____Yes _____No. If yes, please explain:

_____

_____

Please add any additional relevant information about yourself:

_____

_____

Do you agree to background checks as a condition of employment, including employment, criminal, medical, driving and credit?

    _____Yes _____No

References *(Please list two personal and two employment references.)*

Employer_____Phone #_____

Address_____

Name of Supervisor_____

Dates Employed_____Position Held_____
Duties and Responsibilities_____
Reasons for leaving_____

Employer_____Phone #_____
Address_____
Name of Supervisor_____
Dates Employed_____Position Held_____
Duties and Responsibilities_____
Reasons for leaving_____

Personal references
Name_____Relationship_____
Address_____Phone #_____
City/State/Zip _____

Name_____Relationship_____
Address_____Phone #_____
City/State/Zip _____

I, _____*have applied for*
a position as in-home caregiver for an older person.

I hereby respectfully request that you furnish the necessary information and authorize its release without penalty or liability due to an invasion of privacy or civil rights.

Signature of Applicant _____

Witness _____Date _____

INTERVIEW QUESTIONNAIRE

Begin the interview. *What are you currently doing? Why are you looking for work?*_____

_____

_____

Review the application. *How long did you stay on your previous job? What were your responsibilities? How did you get along with your employer? Why did you leave?*_____

_____

_____

Describe the job. (After describing possible challenges and problems, seek the applicant's reactions.) *Do you feel uncomfortable about performing any of these duties or responsibilities?*_____

_____

_____

Stress that good health is mandatory. *How is your health? Have you had a physical exam within the past year, or are you willing to have one done?*_____

_____

_____

Discuss modes of transportation in detail. *What will be your backup system for car trouble or broken-down buses?*_____

_____

_____

Ask open-ended questions. *What made you call our ad? Why does this job appeal to you?*_____

_____

_____

Ask judgement questions. *What would you do if you found the elder lying on the floor?*_____

_____

Conclude the interview. *Do you have any questions?*_____

_____

Broaching the Topic of Theft

It's a good idea to discuss the problem of theft openly and matter-of-factly during the first interview. You could ask, "Would you be willing to take a lie detector test if something were missing?" A knowledgeable applicant may be aware that lie detectors have limited validity and that most private employers are prohibited from requiring job applicants to submit to one. You may have no intention of resorting to such measures, but it makes for an interesting and revealing discussion. An angry or defensive over-reaction on her part may indicate some past problem that you should explore further. It also puts the applicant on the alert that you will take a very hard line when it comes to theft.

Another aspect of the theft issue is accusations. Some elders, particularly if confused or disoriented, hide things for safekeeping, and then can't remember what they've done with the items. They may begin to believe that the items have been stolen and may accuse the caregiver. Other items are legitimately lost, disappearing into the couch, the trash, even the toilet. In any case, you may have to deal with an elder's word against the caregiver's. You might prepare for such an eventuality by asking the applicant how she would handle being accused of stealing by an older person for whom she was caring.

If you are in doubt about the job candidate's trustworthiness, politely put her on notice that you will notify the police should property loss occur. Or, drop a hint that you file the names of home care workers with the police as a precaution against theft. (Check with local police to determine their procedures for such filing.)

More information on theft and other potentially serious problems, including substance abuse and elder abuse, can be found in the next chapter. Just be cognizant during the screening and selecting process of issues involving trustworthiness, emotional health and lifestyle stability. And zero in with laser-intensity if the job candidate gives you hints that her background includes a substance abuse problem or a criminal record. Asking penetrating questions is one effective way to insure that a person with a problem gets the picture that a job with you is not the job for her.

Judging for Yourself

Sometimes your "head" will tell you the job candidate is well qualified but your "heart" tells you "watch out." It may also happen the other way: your "head" is concerned about lack of experience but your "heart" says, "This is a good person." *Listen to both*, and use both the facts and the feelings you get from the interview to help make your selection. Your comfort level with your home caregiver is vital to your success in consumer-directed home care.

Here are some signs that, while not necessarily red flags, should give you pause for thought and trigger further questioning/investigation:

- no work references
- gaps in employment
- frequent moves in and out of state
- no driver's license
- no phone number
- living in area less than one year
- obviously overqualified for the job

Note: Take a look at the vehicle the job seeker drives. Does it appear to be packed with all her worldly belongings? If so, this is an indication that she may have no real home. Sadly, this is a fairly frequent occurence, and a definite "red flag" for you.

FIRST IMPRESSIONS WORKSHEET

_____	_____	Neatly dressed and groomed?
_____	_____	Alert and paying attention?
_____	_____	Friendly, relaxed manner?
_____	_____	Good eye contact?
_____	_____	Physically able?
_____	_____	Good judgment?
_____	_____	Adequately trained?
_____	_____	Wholesome lifestyle?

Checking References

Reference checking can be done either over the telephone or by mail. Of course the telephone is the quickest means (and you may get impressions and/or spontaneous information that you'd never get in writing!). If, however, you choose to use the postal system, be sure to send a self-addressed, stamped envelope to expedite the process. When you call to check work references, ensure the accuracy of all stated information and reasons for resignation. Evaluate any discrepancy between the job seeker's version and the ex-employer's version of past history. Using the sheets as a guide should help you to feel more comfortable about collecting personal information in a systematic and matter-of-fact way.

As for personal references, you may shy away from checking them because it's time consuming and because you are hesitant to invade someone's privacy. It's OK to call! You will be amazed at how helpful others are when it comes to providing assistance relating to home care of frail elders.

Whatever system you choose, mail or phone, don't take shortcuts. This is your opportunity to quiz other people who have known the job candidate. *Verify all information!* Do not make a job offer without checking all references, even if it means writing or calling out of state. Make sure you call *all* the provided names and phone numbers. Ask each for the names and phone numbers of others who know the applicant. If you find that a reference has moved or closed the business, make sure that you obtain a replacement reference from the job applicant.

If you are unable to reach certain individuals, call the applicant and let her know. Ask for work numbers. Try calling at different times during the day.

Following up on both personal and employment references listed on the application should be made easier through the use of the reference check worksheets that follow.

Personal Reference Check Worksheet

Reference name_____

Address_____

Phone number_____

How long have you known this person? Dates? In what relationship?_____

_____

_____

How do you view this person's suitability as a family home helper for an older person?_____

_____

_____

What are her best qualities? Her worst?_____

_____

_____

How does the job seeker get along with others?_____

_____

_____

Do you know her family? Have you ever visited her home?

_____

_____

Are you aware of any problems with drugs or alcohol? Is there anything I should know about her emotional stability, positive or negative?_____

_____

Would the job seeker be a good match for this position? (Describe the job specifics)_____

_____

_____

_____

_____

Thank you very much for providing this information.

EMPLOYMENT REFERENCE CHECK WORKSHEET

Supervisor's Name and Title_____
_____

Company Name_____
Phone #_____

What was the applicant's position, job title and description?
_____
_____

How well did the applicant get along with others?_____
_____
_____

How would you rate the applicant as a worker?_____
_____
_____

What was the applicant's overall job performance? Good
points? Weak points? Attitude?_____
_____
_____

Was the applicant frequently late or absent?_____
_____

Did you find applicant trustworthy? Honest?_____

Were you aware of any substance abuse on the job?_____

Why did applicant leave?_____
_____

Was the worker frequently absent due to health problems?
_____
_____

Would you rehire?_____

Thank you very much for providing this information.

Final Decisions

After a job seeker has been screened, interviewed and has passed satisfactorily through an initial reference check, you should feel ready to make your decision. Get back to the home caregiver that you've decided upon as quickly as possible. Ask if she's still interested and available, then go ahead and offer her the job!

If none of the applicants excites you, *don't pick the best of the worst!* Begin again. You simply may not have interviewed the right person. Or, you may need to change the job description or raise the salary.

Making the Job Offer

- When you are ready to make the job offer, a telephone call, rather than a written note, permits a quick follow-up to the interview.
- Propose a starting wage. Give specific periods of time that reviews/raises will be given.
- Let the candidate know how often she will be paid: daily, weekly or biweekly.
- The offer should be made in such a way that it is *contingent on the receipt of satisfactory background checks* (discussed in the next chapter).
- Allow time for consideration of the offer, but give a date by which you would like a final decision.
- Set a date for the candidate to meet you at your home, sign a contract, sign forms for the release of personal information, and meet the elder.
- Discuss the date of the first day of work.

It's a good idea to call back the other job candidates that you interviewed. Tell them that you've ended your search, and ask if you may keep their name on file for future use:

"Mrs. Lewis, I'm calling to tell you that I have chosen another person for the home caregiver position. I want to thank you for taking the time

and trouble of interviewing with me. Your qualifications are very good, and I'd like to keep your application on file. May I call you in the event of any future job openings? Thank you very much."

Keep a list of the names and addresses of those you don't hire in case your first choice doesn't work out. Also, candidates who took other jobs may know workers whom they can recommend. Be sure to save your completed worksheets, applications, and any other notes you may have taken!

Should You Conduct Background Checks?

Background checks — information about job performance, physical and emotional health, public records, and the general accuracy of information supplied by the prospective employee — may be conducted by telephone, mail or face-to-face interview. Such checks are vital to finding the ideal home caregiver. In fact, you shouldn't allow an employee to start work without first conducting a very thorough one, which may take several weeks. It may be inconvenient to delay the first day on the job for this length of time, but it is highly recommended that you do so. You simply cannot take the risk of allowing a home caregiver into your home until you are thoroughly comfortable with her background profile.

These interim weeks need not be wasted, however. This time can be profitably used for supervised on-the-job training and/or supervised get-acquainted visits with the elder and family. The employee can also get a physical check-up and any necessary medical tests completed during this time.

In the following chapter, we'll take an in-depth look at the process of conducting a thorough background check.

Chapter Six

RUNNING
BACKGROUND CHECKS

"There have been incredible rip-offs. It's the luck of the draw."
— Bruce Hightower
National Academy of Elder Law Attorneys

IT'S TRUE THAT HOME CARE IS THE KEY TO LIVING LONGER and living better in the community. Yet, the isolated privacy of the home care setting opens the door to substandard, unreliable or even abusive treatment. For this reason, thorough background checking is perhaps the most critically important part of the caregiver hiring process. Most professionals who work in this field can relate a worst-case scenario or two involving frail elders and hired helpers, although research data to support the nature or extent of problems are nearly impossible to come by. Rough estimates from Florida suggest that perhaps 25% of all workers who apply for home jobs have criminal records. With thorough and painstaking attention to background checks, however, you certainly do not need to subject yourself to the "luck of the draw," or to those who wish to prey on frail elders.

This chapter lays out the essentials of getting the picture on someone's past — a profile of driving, credit, employment, police and medical records. But before getting into the how's and how-to's of background checks, it's important to discuss briefly the most problematic areas: theft, substance abuse and elder abuse.

Theft

Ninety-five percent of the women who work in home care do so because they have a special caring for older people; a few however are driven by less savory motives. Some may have an inclination toward petty theft; and a tiny minority may be prone to very serious kinds of stealing. One alarming scenario is the employee who must steal to support an expensive drug habit.

Your best protection against criminal activity is the extensive screening, interviewing, and background checking discussed in this book. Also, when it comes to the issue of theft, be careful not to overly tempt human nature by leaving jewelry, cash, credit cards or checkbooks lying carelessly about the house.

Substance Abuse

It has been the experience of some elders that their medication can disappear quickly, especially tranquilizers, pain pills and muscle relaxants. Still others have reported liquor missing. Keeping liquor and medications under lock and key certainly bears consideration.

Experts agree that alcohol and drugs are the roots of a multitude of difficulties, from petty theft, to absenteeism, all the way to financial exploitation and physical abuse. Rather than trying to rehabilitate an employee who is having a problem with potentially addictive substances, focus instead on detecting whether potential employees abuse drugs or alcohol *before* they are hired. One way to screen out the worker with a problem is assertive questioning during the interview process. Another is screening out those who might cause you problems through background checks and/or lab testing. When skillfully done, these two methods nearly always reveal any history of alcoholism or drug abuse.

Physical/Emotional Abuse

Public awareness of the sad and shocking fact of elder abuse has been heightened lately through a good deal of media exposure. We are learning that abuse of elders can manifest itself in a variety of forms, be it physical, psychological or financial. These reports, while unsettling, may actually spur you on to do a more professional job of managing your program of home care. Openness to the potential of abuse in its various forms is a must for those involved in home care.

While helpful, media coverage of elder abuse fails to reveal the true magnitude of this problem, or to identify mechanisms wherein abusers may be identified and screened out *before* they are hired. To address these issues, many states now maintain computerized registries listing those who have been implicated in the abuse of elders. The basic step of screening for a history of abusiveness by obtaining information from these registries is covered later in this chapter.

Are Background Checks Really Necessary?

Your reaction to the foregoing overview of theft, substance abuse and elder abuse may well be one of dismay and discomfort. If so, the case has been made for the importance of conducting thorough background checks. If you remain unconcerned about these issues, your attention is directed to Chapter Eight and the discussion there of supervision of a home caregiver.

No person, agency or book can guarantee that an in-home worker won't harm elders or steal them blind. Caution, even extreme caution, may be the better part of wisdom when it comes to deciding on the time, effort and expense you will invest in background checking. Following the steps outlined in this chapter should give you some peace of mind.

If you've known the worker and/or the worker's family over a period of time, you may already have first-hand knowledge of her background. Or, if she has had a very steady work history for families that have personally recommended her, background checks may seem unnecessary. The decision whether or not to skip the time-consuming background checking process is essentially a personal one, and must be decided on a case-by-case basis.

If you do decide to undertake background checks, it's very important to have the prospective home caregiver sign proper release forms before you proceed. Many agencies require a signed release form, and the release also protects you in the unlikely event that an employee brings suit against you relating to the disclosure of personal information. A sample release form for general purposes can be found on page 79. More specialized release forms that may be needed in a variety of situations are provided throughout this chapter.

The summary on the following page lists the sample forms found in this chapter, each of which is designed to enable you to fulfill your "right to know" without violating the applicant's "right to privacy."

Credit Records

The Fair Credit Reporting Act protects individuals from unauthorized access to their credit records. Although credit records often contain a wealth of sensitive information — including loan defaults, bankruptcies and court judgements — employers are limited to using the information provided only to verify previous employment! (This provision of the law has been likened to asking a jury to disregard the previous question.)

Employers may obtain credit reports directly from credit bureaus once a release is obtained from the prospective employee. Household employers are advised against the do-it-yourself approach in this instance, however. In order to stay within the letter of the detailed and extensive law, the wisest course may be to obtain credit reports through the services of a licensed information broker.

SUMMARY OF BACKGROUND CHECK FORMS

General Release Form (page 79)
Purpose: all purpose
When completed: initial interview
Completed by whom: applicant
Date completed _____

Medical Forms (pages 76-77)
Employee Statement of Health
Purpose: applicant rules out pre-existing health problems
When completed: after signing employment agreement; pending first work day
Completed by whom: applicant
Date completed _____

Medical History Form (page 78)
Purpose: physician rules out pre-existing health problems
When completed: after signing employment agreement; pending first work day
Completed by whom: applicant and physician
Date completed _____

Abuse Records Form (page 83)
Purpose: to rule out abuse history
When completed: after signing employment agreement;
   pending first work day
Completed by whom: applicant and employer
*Date completed*_____

Police Records Form (page 84)
Purpose: to rule out criminal history
When completed: after signing employment agreement;
   pending first work day
Completed by whom: applicant and employer
Date completed _____

General Cover Letter (page 85)
Purpose: all purpose — send with all release forms
When completed: after signing employment agreement;
   pending first work day
Completed by whom: employer
Date completed _____

Driving Records

If a home caregiver will be transporting the elder by car, your first priority is to make sure that she has a valid driver's license. If she does not have a valid driver's license, find out why. It may be because the license was revoked or allowed to lapse. Check the Department of Motor Vehicles' records on lapsed and/or revoked licenses.

A valid license doesn't make someone a good driver, so you need to check on driving records. In many states, you can obtain driving records through the mail with a signed release form. The job candidate will need to supply her full name, her birth date, her driver's license number, and the reason for the request. Additionally, include notarized signatures for the both of you. Send the search request to your state's Department of Motor Vehicles. Typically a search will cost about $3-$5 with a turn-around time of two weeks or more.

The driving record will tell you the "where's and when's" of moving violations, including Driving Under the Influence (DUI). It may also include information on accidents and give the location of each accident.

If driving will be part of the job, it's important to take a test drive with the prospective caregiver. If she'll be using the elder's car, help her to get familiar with its idiosyncrasies. Discuss what action you would want her to take in the event that the car breaks down, where she will be allowed to take the elder in the car, and how she'll be reimbursed for gas.

One good way to structure a test drive is to spontaneously ask a potential home caregiver to give you a lift to the supermarket or other destination. That way, the driver under observation will not be forewarned that you are actually conducting a test of her driving skills and habits.

Medical Records

For your well-being and for that of the employee, you should always require a home caregiver to have a medical examination prior to her first day on the job. This reveals any health condition that needs to be taken into account as you make work assignments. You should pay for both the physical check-up and lab testing to detect any contagious diseases.

TB testing is a must. A skin test for tuberculosis may be obtained from a family physician or at the local health department. The skin test can cost from $5 to $25. If the employee has previously tested positive on a TB test, or does so on the current test, an X-ray will also be required.

HIV, the human immuno-deficiency virus that can lead to AIDS, is a widespread health concern these days. However, HIV has never been shown to be transmitted through the

EMPLOYEE STATEMENT OF HEALTH

1. Have you ever had a serious illness, injury, or operation?
    Yes_____ No_____

    _____

2. Have you ever received Workers' Compensation benefits for
    an injury?   Yes_____ No_____

3. Do you now have, or have you ever had, any disability
    including the following? If so, please circle.
    Epilepsy   Diabetes   Cardiac Disease
    Cerebral Palsy   Vascular Disorder   Parkinson's Disease
    Hemophilia   Hyperinsulinism   Muscular Dystrophy
    Thrombophlebitis   Total Deafness   Mental Retardation
    Multiple Sclerosis   Chronic Osteomyelitis

5   Have you ever had, or do you now have, back trouble or
    complaints? Yes_____ No_____

6. Have you ever had:

    Total loss of sight in one or both eyes, or a partial loss of
    corrected vision of more than 75% bilaterally?
    Yes_____ No_____

    Herniated intervertebral disc?
    Yes_____ No_____

Surgical removal of an intervertebral disc or spinal fusion?
Yes_____ No_____

Residual disability from poliomyelitis?
Yes_____ No_____

Emotional or nervous disorder?
Yes_____ No_____

6. Any permanent physical condition which constitutes a 20% impairment of a member, or of the body as a whole?
Yes_____ No_____

7. Explain all "Yes" answers.

_____

_____

_____

_____

_____

_____

_____

_____

_____

_____

_____

_____   _____
Signature of Employee/Applicant   Date

SPECIAL RELEASE FORM — Medical History

Authorization to Obtain and Disclose Information

I authorize_____to obtain medical information for employment. Any person having such information as to a diagnosis, the treatment, or prognosis of any physical or mental conditions of me, and any non-medical information is authorized to give it to the above parties. The persons authorized to give this information include any doctor, or other health or health-related facility, employer, or insurance company that may have such information.

I am aware that I may obtain a copy of this authorization obtained by the above named individual.

A photocopy of this authorization shall be as effective as the original.

_____At_____

Date

_____

Name of Applicant

Position Description: In-home eldercare provider (Home Caregiver), 20 hours per week or more. Duties may include: some assistance with walking and movement, cooking, cleaning, and driving. Due to the nature of this position, good emotional health is essential. In your opinion is the applicant free of disease or serious mental or emotional handicaps that would be detrimental to the elder with whom the applicant will be working? _____

_____

In your opinion, is the applicant free of physical disabilities that would prevent the performance of the above-mentioned duties?_____

_____

_____   _____

Physician's Signature   *Date*

GENERAL RELEASE FORM — Background Checks

Authorization To Obtain And Disclose Information

I,_____, hereby
authorize _____ to
contact my former employers and references and conduct a
complete background review, including criminal, motor
vehicle and medical. I authorize release and forever discharge
each employer, reference, police, motor vehicle department,
educational institution and medical practice and its employees
and agents from any and all liability of any kind or nature
whatsoever relative to my complete background review. I
further specifically request that all agencies, representatives
and references fully cooperate with this investigation.

If employed, I further authorize periodic checks of all above
referenced sources as may be deemed necessary by employer.

A photocopy of this authorization shall be as effective as the
original.

_____   _____
Job Applicant's Full Name   Signature

_____   _____
Social Security Number   Date

_____
Date of Birth

_____   _____
Driver's License#   State

environment — only blood and other bodily secretions are implicated. Therefore, there is almost no known risk of catching AIDS from an in-home worker providing basic personal care. However, hired caregivers with impaired immune systems are at increased risk of catching severe infections from others.

The question of whether workers infected with HIV can safely be allowed to perform home care duties must be determined on an individual basis. It should be noted, however, that many states treat AIDS as a handicap, and therefore prohibit involuntary AIDS testing or the use of test results to affect employment decisions.

Other than TB testing, the medical examination involves a checkup by a physician. The doctor will be asked to sign a Medical History Form, indicating that he or she is not aware of any contraindicating mental or physical condition.

It's also a good idea to obtain a documented statement of physical condition from the prospective worker herself. Such a statement serves as future insurance against any potential compensation claims by establishing a record of health at the time of employment.

The Employee Statement of Health sample on pages 76-77 is similar to those that home health agencies require of job applicants.

Information Brokers

Research companies and independent information brokers have perfected the art of quickly running background checks. For a fee, they will access nationwide computerized databases to track down the details of an individual's credit history, driving record, possible criminal record, employment history and numerous other bits of information.

Hiring an expert to do the critically important work of background checking for you is certainly an option. There are many companies that specialize in checking out the backgrounds of job applicants.

At this writing, in Florida, $100 will purchase a basic pre-employment background check by an information broker, a licensed investigator or an employment consultant. Check the Yellow Pages for listings under these or similar categories.

Abuse Registries

Some states maintain special databases on those individuals on whom a report of elder abuse or neglect has been confirmed. Call the state-funded social services department in your area to inquire if such information is available to employers, and, if so, how it may be obtained.

Usually, if a substantiated report of elder abuse is on file with the state, you will receive a brief written notice. This will give the victim's name, the perpetrator's name, and the date when the record of abuse was filed. Of course, the existence of such a report would immediately disqualify anyone from employment as a home caregiver.

If no record is found, you will also receive a notice of a clean record in regard to elder abuse.

Arrest Records

It may be possible, in some communities, to obtain local arrest records. This information may even be provided over the phone if you can provide a full name, birth date, and social security number. In some localities you will need a signed release to initiate a records search — in this case, you may deal with the law enforcement agency by mail. In other communities, access to arrest records will be strictly limited. In California, for example, even law enforcement agencies must have a valid criminal case pending in order to access such records.

Begin by calling the local police department or Sheriff's office to inquire as to the proper procedure for obtaining a check of arrest records.

As for state records, call the state law enforcement or criminal records department to determine the correct procedure. In Florida, for instance, it takes about two weeks and costs $15 to learn if a person has been convicted for drug possession, assault, robbery, rape or murder in the state. The Florida Department of Law Enforcement will also conduct national searches at $15 for each report.

In cases where a criminal record is revealed, but it was not a felony or a first-degree misdemeanor, your family must make the determination whether or not the conviction precludes the worker from employment as a home caregiver. A person convicted of a felony or first-degree misdemeanor is *never* appropriate for employment that involves the personal care of dependent persons.

Procedures and fees for such law enforcement checks vary by state and community, and are subject to change as laws are changed. Check with local officials to determine current availability and costs where you live.

Note: A criminal records check is always advisable when hiring home caregivers. Such a check is not foolproof, however. For certain offenses, individuals are able to escape detection by having their criminal records "expunged."

SPECIAL RELEASE FORM
ABUSE OF ELDERLY

_____
Date

Applicant_____
(job applicant's name)

    I hereby authorize the prospective employer named below to make inquiry of any central abuse registry in regard to the existence of any report of abuse, neglect or exploitation of the elderly (or of any person) in which I may have been involved, and to release the results of that investigation to such prospective employer.

_____   _____
Job Applicant's Signature   Date

_____
Job Applicant's Name (last name, first name, middle name)

_____
Maiden Name

_____
Prior Name(s)

_____ _____   _____
Gender   Date of Birth   Social Security #

_____
Job Applicant's Present Address (include dates of residence)
Job Applicant's Previous Addresses (include dates)

1. _____
2. _____
3. _____
Employer requesting background check:

Name_____Phone#_____

_____
Street Address

_____
City   County   State   Zip

SPECIAL RELEASE FORM
POLICE RECORDS

Waiver of Liability and Release of Claims

I hereby authorize the_____
Police Department to release any information it may have in its records or may obtain from other sources under my name and birth date, including my fingerprints, to_____
_____ and I hereby release and forever discharge the_____Police Department and its agents, officers, and employees from any and all actions, causes of actions, claims and demands for, upon or by any reason for any damage, loss or injury, which may be sustained by me in the nature of libel, slander, invasion of privacy or other results from errors or omissions in the information given or from the use of the information, whether by reason or unauthorized use, negligence or otherwise.

Name_____

Address_____

_____

Date of Birth_____

State of_____

County of_____

A photocopy of this authorization shall be as valuable as the original.

Employer requesting background check:

Name_____   Phone_____

_____
Street Address   City   Zip   County

GENERAL RELEASE COVER LETTER

(Use this cover letter with the Background Checks General Release Form found on page 79 or with the other varieties of release forms found on pages 78, 83 and/or 84.))

Date:

Attention:

Sir/Madame:

Enclosed is a letter of authorization from a candidate seeking employment with me as a in-home personal care worker. Prior to employment I want to do everything possible to check the person's background thoroughly as the employee will be working in close contact with a frail older person. One way of doing this is to request your department to check the applicant's record.

Would you please send a copy of your findings to me at the address below?

Thank you very much for your cooperation and attention to my request.

Employer's Name_____

Address_____

Phone_____

_____
Employer's Signature

Chapter Seven

COMPLETING THE EMPLOYMENT AGREEMENT

"Anna cared for my wife of thirty-eight years each day. Nothing was any problem for her. She was always cheerful and doing more than was expected, even though she had some heartaches of her own.

My wife passed away recently from her long illness — we'll never forget our Anna. She did so much to help my wife in her hours of need."
— Bill Clarkson, spouse/caregiver, age 72

HOME CARE BY ITS VERY DEFINITION INVOLVES HUMAN relationships. Legal issues always present a stark contrast to the gentler aspects of this very personal enterprise. But they weave their way through many of the steps of hiring a home caregiver and, as unappealing as written agreements and labor laws may seem, every employer must come to terms with them.

It's important to establish the ground rules of employment early on, clarifying expectations on both sides and spelling out duties to be performed, hours to be worked, compensation, time off and other details. An employment agreement should reflect the desires, needs and wishes of the elder and family when it comes to the plan of care.

The sample agreement in this chapter can be used as a model when writing your own. You may elect to add more or to leave some things out, tailoring your particular document to suit your needs. *Note: The form provided in this book is not intended to serve in place of legal advice.* If you have any questions about the legal consequences of writing this type of document, you should consult an attorney in your area who specializes in federal and state labor law. And remember, once an applicant is offered the job and accepts, the agreement should be signed before the worker starts. Both the caregiver and the family representative should retain a copy of the signed agreement.

Following the "Sample Employment Agreement" you'll find a summary description and explanation of each of its elements. The chapter concludes with some tools that will help you develop a job description and evaluate your employee.

SAMPLE EMPLOYMENT AGREEMENT

This agreement between:_____
(hereinafter referred to as Caregiver)

and_____
(hereinafter referred to as Family)

is intended to clarify specific working conditions and terms of employment, and to set guidelines for the Caregiver to follow at all times while

_____

a member of the Family, is in her care.

1. Work Schedule
   The Helper's daily work schedule will be as follows:
   Monday_____to _____
   Tuesday_____to _____
   Wednesday_____to _____
   Thursday_____to _____
   Friday_____to _____
   Saturday_____to _____
   Sunday_____to _____
   Total weekly hours_____

2. Time Off
   The Helper will be off, but unpaid for the following holidays:

_____
_____

   _____weeks of unpaid vacation may be taken during the first year on the job. After the first year, paid vacation will be earned in accordance with total time worked. Vacation dates will be set by mutual agreement between the Family and Caregiver.

3. Compensation
The Family agrees to pay the Caregiver $_____ per, _____ as gross wages. The Family will withhold and remit to appropriate agencies all Federal, State and Local taxes,

as well as Workers Compensation. A W2 statement will be supplied to the Caregiver by January 31 for the previous calendar year.

In the event the Family seeks the services of the Caregiver for additional services, she will be paid at a rate to be determined on a job-by-job basis.

4. Performance Reviews and Pay Increases

Performance reviews will be given once each _____. A merit pay increase may follow a performance review, but there can be no guarantee of an increase. Merit increases will not be given if the Caregiver's performance is not satisfactory.

5. Car Use

The family agrees to pay gasoline mileage at a rate of $_____ per mile for use of the Caregiver's car when authorized by the Family as necessary for carrying out the care responsibilities under this agreement. The Caregiver agrees to keep an accurate log of these miles. The Caregiver agrees to abide by all the laws of the State of _____, including the proper use of seat belts at all times. The Caregiver agrees to provide the Family with proof of adequate auto insurance on her own vehicle or, if the car is supplied by the Family, the Family will provide the Caregiver with proof of insurance coverage for both the Caregiver and the car. The Caregiver's travel from home to work and back again, or to other assignments, will not be reimbursed.

6. Meals

The Family will_____ / will not_____ pay for the Caregiver's on-the-job meals during the work assignment.

7. Work Rules

Verbal or physical abuse is grounds for dismissal.
Alcohol or drug use on the job is grounds for dismissal.
Reporting to work intoxicated is grounds for dismissal.
Smoking is prohibited in the house or in the car.

Personal phone calls (local or long distance toll calls) are not permitted.

Coming to work late is grounds for dismissal.

number of absences to result in termination_____

number of tardinesses to result in termination_____

Visitors are not permitted during the work period.

Gifts — the giving and taking of gifts, money, or other exchanges between the Caregiver and older member of the family is not allowed.

8. Termination

The Family and Caregiver agree that the Family has the right to terminate the Caregiver's employment at any time, for any reason, or without a reason. Prior notification is not necessary under the terms of this agreement.

Likewise, the Caregiver may terminate his/her employment at will.

We agree to these terms of employment.

Caregiver

_____Date:_____
                 signature

Authorized Representative(s) of the Family

_____ Date:_____

_____ Date:_____
                 signature

Work Scheduling, Time Off and Back-up Help

Elders often need help for short periods of time in the early morning, evenings and on the weekends. Flexibility of scheduling is one of the advantages of consumer-directed home care. For instance, the home caregiver's schedule can be dovetailed with those of others who may also be filling in to provide the necessary level of care. The elder may receive visits daily or several times a week; she may need services only a couple of hours per visit, all day, or at times, day and night. Services may last several weeks, months or years.

It is a common mistake for the elder and family to rely solely upon one home caregiver with no allowances for the possibility of her becoming ill, developing transportation problems, getting weathered-in, experiencing some other type of difficulty or wishing to take a vacation. Although adequate notice for time off or leaving the job should be negotiated at the time of hire, there are occasions when prior notice cannot be given. For these situations, it is imperative that you have a back-up plan in place.

Home health agencies are prime sources of nurse's aides and homemakers/home health aides for back-up help. These personnel are usually available on short notice. Another possibility is nursing homes that might be willing to refer aides who want to earn extra money during their off-duty hours. It's a good idea to keep a running list of names and telephone numbers of people who might be available for work on short notice. Or, you might ask your home caregiver if she has her own substitute. It's worth asking!

Back-up helpers may be former employees, applicants who were not hired but were successfully screened, family members, and friends. You may wish to have these people come in one or two days in advance of need to familiarize them with your routine. Visiting nurses and home health agencies can also be called upon, but their services are likely to be expensive. Some community agencies may provide limited back-up services as well; check your local Yellow Pages (under "Senior Citizen Services") for programs in your community.

It is also absolutely essential that you arrange for regular periods of relief and vacation for the home caregiver. Regardless of her devotion and competence, the care of elders brings its share of demands, frustration, and stress. To provide a break from the routine, friends or relatives may be willing to take over at regular intervals, or you may need to hire a temporary, part-time replacement.

Some families employ more than one home caregiver at a time. For example, Mrs. M has one helper who works mornings and one who works evenings. If one home caregiver is unable to work, the other may be able to fill in.

A sample time card is found at the end of this chapter. Even if your home caregiver's schedule does not vary from week to week, it's a good idea to complete the card for each week worked. The accumulated cards will help you when it comes to calculating annual Social Security taxes. If your caregiver's hours are irregular, the time card will record exactly the amount due each week for services rendered.

Compensation, Taxes, and Benefits

Home care workers are generally paid at, or just above, the minimum hourly wage; and they sometimes quit because they want higher salaries. You may boost the competitiveness of your job compared to similar ones available through home care agencies if you're able to pay higher wages. For instance, if a home health agency in town pays $5.50 an hour, you might pay $6.00 or $6.50 an hour. *Paying just a little more per hour has shown to significantly lengthen the time a home helper will stay in your employment before moving on.*

You may be tempted to pay your home caregiver in cash in an under-the-table arrangement. This scenario is appealing because it appears that you could avoid filling out forms and paying taxes (see Chapter Ten). Unfortunately, it's illegal. If caught, you face embarrassment and stiff penalties.

Always pay your helper by check. Use receipt forms or some form of written proof that you made payments to your employee. Generic receipt books, which are available at office supply and stationery stores, work well for this purpose.

In-home caregivers working more than eight hours per week on a regular basis are considered employees and must be paid minimum wage in accordance with federal law. As the employer, you assume responsibility for Social Security (FICA) and Federal Unemployment (FUTA) taxes. Where the consumer is the employer, worker's compensation coverage is not mandated by federal law. Some states, however, require you to pay state taxes and worker's compensation. More on this in Chapter Ten.

Workers in consumer-directed home care rarely receive more than limited benefits of employer contributions to Social Security. Offering your home caregiver some benefits beyond those required, however, will give her the satisfaction of knowing that you are trying to address her needs.

You may wish to try one or more of these incentives:

- Merit pay increases are an excellent way to recognize and reinforce a job well done. They are not given automatically, but are based on satisfactory performance. (Be careful not to give your caregiver reason to expect that she will get a raise with each review.)
- Bonuses — one-time payments — may be given as appropriate for a job well done, to commemorate a special occasion or holiday, or to commend an employee for longevity in employment with your family.

- Shift differentials may be paid to home caregivers who work undesirable hours (evenings, nights, and weekends), or agree to serve on an on-call basis.
- Reimbursement for bus or other transit passes.
- Mileage or expense reimbursement for worker driving her own car.
- Partial salary for time spent in transit.
- One paid day off for six months perfect attendance.
- Bonus of $.50/hour for no missed time for one month.
- Payment to attend special training classes.

Car Use

When it comes to home caregivers transporting elders, you have basically three options:

Car Option #1: The caregiver transports the elder in the elder's *car.* Note: The owner of the vehicle is responsible for the negligence of any driver. If the home caregiver uses the family car, you will be responsible for any liabilities that she incurs.

Be sure to add the home caregiver as a driver on the auto insurance policy that covers the elder's vehicle. You may wish to investigate the purchase of an "umbrella liability" insurance policy which will pick up where your auto insurance leaves off. Such a policy can usually be purchased at a small annual cost; a million dollars in coverage costs less than $150 at this writing.

Car Use Option #2: The caregiver transports the elder in her own car. You must make sure that the home caregiver's auto policy provides adequate coverage for the passenger, in this case the older person, in the event of injury in an accident. Be sure to review the home caregiver's auto insurance policy to determine if the liability limits are adequate.

Car Use Option #3: The caregiver provides escort rather than transport services. In situations where you'd like help with transportation and errands, but you wish to sidestep the potential complications associated with the previous two options, consider using your caregiver to *escort* rather than *transport*. With this option, the car used would be a taxicab, a city bus, or a senior services mini-van. The driving would be left to someone else — someone who most assuredly has both a chauffeur's license and full insurance coverage.

With this option, cab or bus fare is supplied by the elder; all the preparation for, and supervision of, the outing is the responsibility of the home caregiver. Unless you have written assurance from an expert that adequate insurance coverage is available in options #1 and #2, you are tempting fate to consider anything other than the escort option.

Meals
As home caregivers do not leave the work site for meals, it's traditional for the elder and family to share meals with them. Your worker may prefer to bring her own meal to store in the refrigerator, and/or eat where and when she chooses. This is permissible as long as she doesn't leave the premises.

Work Rules
Most work rules are just common sense ways to ward off potential problems before they happen. The prohibition against gift taking and giving is slightly out of the ordinary, however. Commercial agencies do not allow employees to accept gifts, money, household goods, and so on, no matter how small. Gift-giving, particularly in the case of elders who may be disoriented, confused, and/or vulnerable and easily intimidated, can become a sore spot. Experience has shown that it is sometimes difficult to tell where generosity ends and "taking advantage" begins. In spite of the goodwill that usually fuels the exchange of gifts, when it comes to frail elders in the home setting, it's a gesture that should be prohibited.

If your home caregiver smokes, and you are concerned about the health hazards to your elder (as you should be), or you simply do not like the smell of a smoky house, consider how you can work this out. A home caregiver could go outside to smoke in good weather, but what about cold weather? Don't compromise too easily. Many work sites are now "smoke free" due to employer mandates. It's not too much to ask that an employee reserve her smoking habits for her own time and her own space.

Similarly, punctuality must be stressed. Of course, at times delays are unavoidable. The home caregiver should be instructed that if a delay occurs, she should telephone to say that she will be late.

As for using the elder's phone for personal calls, exceptions will have to be made from time to time to the "no phone" rule. Permission should always be requested in advance, however, for local calls; long distance calls should not be made by the home caregiver.

Finally, experience has proved that, if a home caregiver is allowed to bring along other people to her job, she will be kept from getting her work done. Adherence to the "no visitors" house rule is strongly advised.

Termination

The "Sample Employment Agreement" specifically gives the Family the right to terminate the Caregiver's employment at any time, for any reason, or for no reason at all. This concept is termed "employment at will," and is designed to avoid possible legal action for "wrongful termination."

Although these terms do not require the employer to explain to the employee the "whys and wherefores" surrounding termination, most employment professionals agree that it is good practice — as well as common courtesy — to do so. How and what you say during a termination transaction, however, is a delicate issue, more fully discussed in Chapter Eight (supervising).

If you wish to offer an explanation for termination, keep in mind that an employer is generally conceded the right to terminate an employee without notice for breaking any of the "house rules," or for more serious offenses such as theft, verbal or physical abuse, intoxication on the job, chronic absences or tardiness, or failure to carry out assigned duties as outlined in the job description.

It is critically important to handle dismissal in the most businesslike way. Start looking for a replacement right away, even if you have given notice; your employee may decide to leave immediately.

More information on the unlovely art of terminating employment agreements can be found in Chapter Eight.

Elder Law Attorneys

A good elder law attorney can help you negotiate a sound employment agreement with your caregiver. Additionally, attorneys who practice elder law, or focus upon the legal needs of persons aged sixty and over, are particularly skilled in helping families and elders plan for the many different aspects of long term care including:

- estate planning/living trusts
- incapacity planning (living wills, health care surrogate, pre-need guardianship)
- benefits eligibility (Medicare/Medicaid/Social Security, pension rights, etc.)
- evaluating long term care insurance coverage
- senior housing contracts (nursing home, low income housing, CCRCs)

To locate an elder law attorney in your community, contact the National Academy of Elder Law Attorneys. Their address and phone number are listed in Appendix G.

Job Description

Now that you have clearly established the conditions of employment, you are ready to hammer out a job description, and/or care plan. This document can serve as a checklist of the caregiver's duties and responsibilities and can be posted in the home as a guide. Also, you, the employer, can use it to evaluate performance on the job. The job description and performance rating forms (samples follow), are tools you will be using during regularly scheduled performance reviews with your home caregiver.

Remember that hiring a person does not mean that you must stay with her for life. If you find that over a period of time your caregiver is incompatible with your needs, you have the power to remove that individual from your employment and start your hiring process again. Your documents are not cast in concrete either. Update your agreement and job description periodically as needed.

* * * * * *

A Point to Consider

An especially crucial aspect of the consumer-directed model of home care is making sure that the rights of both the home care employer and of the home care worker herself are protected. Being among the lowest paid, least benefitted and least visible of American workers, perhaps it is the home caregiver, rather than the employer, who is most at risk. An employment agreement is designed to strengthen and support her options, as well as those of the employer.

CAREGIVER JOB DESCRIPTION*

Bathing_____

Dressing_____

Helping to Bathroom_____

Incontinence Care_____

Mobility_____

Exercise_____

Preparation of Meals_____

Housekeeping_____

Laundry_____

Transportation_____

Grocery shopping_____

Correspondence_____

Other Assistance_____

_____

_____

_____

_____

_____

Employers: Write in a brief description of each.

CARE PLAN

	Monthly	Weekly	Daily	As Needed
Personal Care				
Feed (by hand)	____	____	____	____
Feed (cut food, place utensils, etc.)	____	____	____	____
Feeding supervision (encourage to eat)	____	____	____	____
Assist with bathing (tub, sink or in bed)	____	____	____	____
Wash hair	____	____	____	____
Comb hair	____	____	____	____
Shave	____	____	____	____
Denture care	____	____	____	____
Dress/undress	____	____	____	____
Assist with toileting	____	____	____	____
Assist with moving	____	____	____	____
Meals				
Prepare/serve breakfast	____	____	____	____
Prepare/serve lunch	____	____	____	____
Prepare/serve dinner	____	____	____	____
Prepare special diets	____	____	____	____
Plan meals	____	____	____	____
Laundry				
Wash and dry clothes	____	____	____	____
Fold/put away clothes	____	____	____	____
Other Tasks				
Transport	____	____	____	____
Escort	____	____	____	____

	Monthly	Weekly	Daily	As Needed
Buy personal items and medicines	____	____	____	____
Grocery shopping	____	____	____	____
Housekeeping				
Clean floor	____	____	____	____
Clean bathroom/ kitchen fixtures and appliances	____	____	____	____
Dust furniture and pick up clutter	____	____	____	____
Wash and dry dishes	____	____	____	____
Change bed covers	____	____	____	____
Straighten bed covers	____	____	____	____
Dispose of trash/ garbage	____	____	____	____

PERFORMANCE RATING

Employee's name_____

Family Representative's name_____

Date_____

	Yes	No
Attendance		
Does the caregiver report to work on time and when scheduled?	_____	_____
When caregiver is late or absent, is prior notice given?	_____	_____
Is a valid reason given for lateness/absence?	_____	_____
Performance		
Does caregiver perform duties to elder's and family's satisfaction?	_____	_____
Does caregiver follow instructions well?	_____	_____
Initiative		
Does caregiver work without constant supervision?	_____	_____
Does caregiver steadily and consistently perform her duties?	_____	_____
Attitude and Behavior		
Is the caregiver trustworthy?	_____	_____
Is the caregiver courteous in speech and manner?	_____	_____
Is the caregiver not just competent, but caring?	_____	_____

If you want the best care, nothing short of "yes" to all of the questions above should satisfy you. These are the basics you should expect — and get — in any home care situation.

TIME CARD

Employee's name_____

For the Week of_____ to _____

DAY	HOURS	TOTAL HOURS
Monday	__:__to __:__	_____
Tuesday	__:__to __:__	_____
Wednesday	__:__to __:__	_____
Thursday	__:__to __:__	_____
Friday	__:__to __:__	_____
Saturday	__:__to __:__	_____
Sunday	__:__to __:__	_____

TOTALS FOR WEEK

____hours worked x $_____/hour = total wages of $_____

Deductions from wages $_____

Total paid this pay period $_____

Date check written_____

Check number_____

Chapter Eight

SUPERVISING YOUR CAREGIVER

"You can start good supervision by developing a bee-like set of very sensitive antennae. This will be your early warning system for problems in performance, and also excellence in performance."

— Dorothy Workman, Community Care Program

BECAUSE OF OUR "DO IT YOURSELF" TRADITION ON THE home-front, most Americans have had little experience overseeing in-home workers. Supervision of an employee can seem to be one of the most frustrating and difficult aspects of consumer-directed home care. Rather than developing these highly learnable skills ourselves, most of us have been only too happy to turn the responsibility over to some agency, business or institution.

Obviously home caregivers who provide dependable, efficient service for an older person can make a major difference in that person's ability to live independently. If you elect to "do it yourself," the key to getting high quality service lies with your own supervisory skills. You must create an environment in which the very best personal and job-related traits of your home caregiver can flourish.

You can obtain what you want — the very best in home care — by giving a home caregiver what she wants — a satisfying and rewarding work environment. A true win-win situation! Good supervision begins with orientation and training sessions, conducted before the caregiver's first day on the job.

Orientation and Training

If the elder has been involved in the screening and interviewing of the home caregiver, there may be no need of a special introductory meeting. But, if the older person and caregiver have not yet met, you should schedule a "dress rehearsal" prior to the first day of work. This will serve as the first face-to-face meeting between the home helper and the elder.

Think about the best way to set up this meeting — something as simple as serving coffee in the elder's home might do. This meeting begins the delicate process of relationship-building. Remember, however, that relationships take time, effort and patience. You might anticipate a thawing-out process as the elder warms up to her new caregiver.

Next, have the home caregiver come for an initial orientation/training session before her first day on the job. (Plan to pay the caregiver for this session as you would for a regular work day.) Get home care off to a good start by introducing the caregiver to the elder's home instead of leaving her alone, forced to find her way around. Begin by giving her a tour of the house with the elder present. Briefly explain the layout of rooms and where essential items can be found. Explain how to operate household appliances, air conditioning and heating units, door locks, and so on.

Step-by-step demonstration sessions are the best way to let the new employee see exactly what you require. Discuss your needs in detail, demonstrating the particular way in which you would like things done. Use the "Care Plan" and the "Job

Description" in the previous chapter as guides to outlining the responsibilities of the job.

Help make the caregiver's job easier by letting her know of any special routines or preferences you may have. What may be second nature to you may be second guessing to her. If you consider certain household areas off bounds, say so. Home care should complement an elder's lifestyle as much as possible, so don't be timid about making your wishes known.

Provide the caregiver with the "Elder Information Form" and "Emergency Telephone Numbers" form at the end of this chapter. Go over these in detail with her. These provide her with a written reference sheet of all the information that she will need in case of an emergency. Don't assume that the home caregiver will know what to do in an emergency. *Discuss emergency routines in detail.* For instance, under what circumstances will the home caregiver rush the elder to a hospital, call an ambulance, or call a family member?

Don't expect too much, too soon. A new job is stressful for everyone, perhaps especially so for the caregiver. When it comes to home care, allow for an adjustment period. It may take days or weeks for everyone involved to get comfortable.

After orientation and training, you must focus your full attention upon establishing a work setting that is conducive to productivity and job satisfaction. One of the most unsettling aspects of home care is the high turnover rate. Some families have been lucky enough to find the ideal home caregiver on the first try and to keep her for many years. Other families experience the revolving door syndrome of a seemingly endless stream of short-term helpers who come, work for a few weeks or months, then quit.

You've invested a great deal of time and energy in recruiting and selecting your caregiver. Don't walk away now. Plan to spend lots of time during the first few weeks she's on the job, helping the elder and caregiver to establish a comfortable and effective working relationship. You'll markedly increase the likelihood of success, and you'll keep your carefully selected employee longer!

What Do Home Caregivers Want?

Perhaps the secret of worker retention lies in understanding what home caregivers are looking for in a job and in an employer.

In answering the question, "What Do Home Caregivers Want?", it may come as a surprise to learn that, when given the opportunity to prioritize, workers place good wages toward the bottom of the list! Here are the rank-ordered results of an informal survey of workers taken recently in Florida:

- Feeling "in on things"
- Tactful discipline
- Understanding attitude
- Appreciation
- Good working conditions
- Good wages
- Loyalty from employer

In the rest of this chapter, we'll take a closer look at each of these aspects of the work environment.

Feeling "In On Things"

Feeling "in on things" is the difference between feeling, on the one hand, like a valued employee, and on the other, like plain hired help. The best way to make sure that your home helper feels important and included is by regularly seeking out her insights and opinions.

One good way to accomplish this is to request that your home helper keep a log book. Entries don't have to be lengthy, they can simply reflect the elder's daily moods or feelings: "didn't finish lunch—said she wasn't hungry," "in good mood today," "had difficulty in getting him to dress." The notes in the log book can serve as a summation, and a good reference, for daily or weekly conferences between you and your home caregiver.

Paying the home helper for her time spent in conference with you is a good way to promote exchange of information and increase worker morale at the same time. Home care work, by its very nature, is isolating; you can increase job satisfaction for your caregiver by making it a part of the job to meet regularly with an interested and concerned member of the family. These conferences will give the employee a chance to communicate her needs or grievances to you, and for you to see if she is satisfied with her job and her relationship with your family.

A home caregiver is someone very significant to the well-being of your family and, as such, is much more important than "hired help." Give her the respect and attention that she deserves. With sensitive treatment, the best home caregivers will respond in-kind with dedicated, responsible and enthusiastic care that goes far beyond "an hour's work for an hour's pay."

Tactful Discipline

Everyone appreciates being told when they are doing a good job, but it is also necessary at times to talk about mediocre or poor performance. Its no secret that the small annoyances can cause large problems when swept under the rug. Tactful discipline is an essential component in a good working relationship.

Tactful discipline involves discussing performance problems in a friendly manner, out of the presence of others, and indicating why you are concerned, without anger or accusations. Tactful discipline is sensitive discipline which recognizes that, nine times out of ten, people are doing the best they can. They'd like to do better, and they are willing to try, but they want to "save face" at the same time.

It all boils down to kindness, fairness and being very specific about the behavior you'd like to see changed. An effective technique is for you and your employee to tackle the problem *together*. After discussing both sides of the story, devise a solution (again, together) that works for both of you.

Understanding Attitude

Women take on home caregiver jobs for common-sense reasons. Other than liking older people, the job usually offers an attractive, self-paced workload that might be hard to find in more traditional work settings. For example, a worker may want to arrange her hours so that they won't interfere with leisure or family activities. Younger workers may need job flexibility to attend to small children coming home from school, or to complete coursework at college.

An understanding attitude is flexible, creative and forgiving. An understanding attitude is also one that allows the other party to wear clothes that she's most comfortable in, to set her own pace on the job, and to occasionally make minor mistakes without serious recrimination. After all, although you may need a miracle worker, your home caregiver is only human.

Appreciation

You've got to let your worker know what she means to your family. Certainly, one easy and very effective way to do this is simply to tell her: "You are a lifesaver. I simply don't know what we'd do without you."

Knowing that we make a positive difference in another person's life keeps many of us motivated, despite modest wages. Testimonials from currently-employed workers about the value of feeling appreciated, needed and wanted strongly support this principle.

One simple way to show appreciation is to remember your home caregiver's birthday with a card or present. Another is to treat her to lunch occasionally as an expression of thanks for providing excellent care. There are many ways to recognize valuable work; you might ask the caregiver to offer her own suggestions.

Good Working Conditions

It's your responsibility to provide a work setting, free from hazards, adequate food and supplies, and provisions for emergencies. If a home caregiver is injured because of unsafe equipment or surroundings, she may seek to recover damages. More on this in Chapter Ten.

Training in basic home care skills can be another important ingredient of good working conditions. Consider footing the bill for your helper to attend some special classes. In addition to adding to her technical skills, class attendance allows a caregiver to get to know others working in the field, increasing her identification with her chosen occupation.

Good Wages

The basic requirement of a living wage is regularly disregarded in the field of home care. Many workers are paid minimum wage (less than they could earn at a local fast-food restaurant) and are paid only for the hours actually spent in the home, with no consideration for the hours traveling from one home to another.

If you follow carefully the guidance and strategies presented in this book, you'll be paying your home caregiver wages that are higher than those she could earn performing similar work through an agency.

Loyalty from Employer

Loyalty could be interpreted both as job security and as an employer who recognizes when performance falls into the "above and beyond the call of duty" category. That is, if you've found an excellent home caregiver, you've got to stand by her. This may mean juggling schedules to provide her with sick leave, and/or vacation time. It could mean discussing a plan of raising her wages over time. Loyalty says, "We're all in this together, for the long haul. I'll treat you with fairness and respect, and in return, you'll provide my relative/friend with the very best care." Loyalty says, "None of us are perfect. When I'm displeased, I'll let you know. And when I'm pleased, I'll let you know that, also."

How To Give Feedback

"Feedback" is the heart of good supervision. It is a special kind of ongoing responsiveness from you that will tell the worker how you want the job done. There are four kinds of feedback: positive, corrective, mixed and negative. The home caregiver cannot read your mind; if you strive to communicate your wishes through one of these ways of providing feedback, she's much more likely to respond the way you want her to.

Positive Feedback

Positive feedback reinforces performance.

In order for feedback to be positive it must:

- Praise correct performance.
- Be sincere.
- Describe the situation or behavior that you liked.

Good Examples:

"Mother's hair looks so clean. You really did a great job of washing it today. Thanks for the good shampoo."

"I really appreciate the extra care you take in cleaning under the sofa and bed. Having a clean home is important to Mother."

Bad Examples (non-specific feedback):
"You did a good job."
"Thank you."

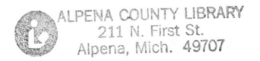

Corrective Feedback

Corrective feedback improves substandard performance. In order for feedback to be corrective it must:

- Specify exactly what action was done incorrectly.
- Give specific instructions for correcting the action.
- Criticize the action, not the employee herself.

Good Examples:

"We need to work on washing mother's hair. I really prefer two washes and a rinse, followed by conditioner."

"The beans at lunch today were a little overcooked. I've found if you cook them on medium for 30 minutes they come out just the way Mother likes them."

Bad Examples:

"Mother's hair looks and feels horrible today."

"You just didn't do it right."

Mixed Feedback

Mixed feedback, like corrective feedback, is designed to improve performance. This technique "sweetens" corrective feedback by mixing it with a little positive feedback. ("A spoonful of sugar helps the medicine go down.") Mixed feedback involves "three pluses and a wish." For example, "I really appreciate having the laundry done so well. You also do such a good job with the dusting and vacuuming. I do wish you would save time to clean the dishes after lunch" — three positive comments and one wish.

While positive, corrective and mixed feedback can be used in most situations, there may be times when the caregiver needs to be corrected more sternly. For example, when the helper continually incorrectly performs tasks that she knows how to do, or when the caregiver tests the family and elder to see what he/she can get away with, negative feedback is required.

Negative Feedback

Negative feedback reprimands the helper. Negative feedback should:

- Be given immediately.
- Be given in a calm tone of voice.
- Specify what was done wrong.
- Spell out the consequences of the action and how upset you are.
- Tell what you expect in the future.

Good Example

"Tina, this is the second day in a row that you have been late with no good excuse. I'm not happy with this pattern. Please don't let this become a habit. I expect you to be on time. If you aren't, I will dock your pay for the time that you miss."

Giving negative feedback effectively is very difficult for most of us. The secret is to give it early, or as soon as the problem comes to your attention. If you let the problem behavior go on for a long time without saying anything, you will find it nearly impossible to give negative feedback without losing your temper. And, that is not good for you or for your worker. Even when giving negative feedback, the idea is to shape problematic behavior into positive behavior, without punishing or damaging the employee's self-esteem. Once the negative feedback is given, forgive and forget.

Timing of Feedback

Studies have shown that it's not only what you say, but *how and when you say it.* If you can master the types and timing of feedback, you are well on your way to becoming an effective supervisor. And, your home caregiver will appreciate you for it.

Try to remember the S.O.S. of feedback:

S Soon   *Give feedback immediately after a problem occurs.*

O One   *Give feedback on only one incident at a time.*

S Short   *Keep feedback short and to the point.*

Disciplining Your Caregiver

Disciplining moves beyond negative feedback, starting out where the latter ends. Discipline is a labor-intensive process, and should only be undertaken if you believe that the home helper can learn from her mistakes, and is willing to mend her ways. Typically, complaints about in-home workers fall into three categories:

- *Absenteeism:* lateness, prolonged lunch breaks, leaving early, or frequent absences.
- *Misconduct:* breaking rules as outlined in the Employment Agreement, i.e., smoking, using foul language, frequent phone use, etc.
- *Poor Performance:* poor attitude, underperformance (just getting by) or incorrect performance.
  Note: "Poor performance" includes any pattern of rough, indifferent, or careless caregiving.

Workers can correct their personal habits; however an indifferent attitude or a rough style of care are not easily changed.

Types of Disciplinary Action

A *written notice of unsatisfactory performance* reinforces verbal negative feedback. It warns the caregiver in writing and places her on notice as to an impending dismissal if her performance doesn't improve. Giving the home caregiver a copy of the "Notice of Unsatisfactory Performance" (included at the end of this chapter) will reinforce what was discussed during a face-to-face meeting with her.

This unfortunate situation is a very unpleasant aspect of consumer-directed home care. Dismissal may be appropriate for the first serious offense, or as the final step in progressive discipline that has involved prior notice of unsatisfactory performance. Dismissal may follow an unsatisfactory performance review, or it may occur due to an infraction of one or more of the "Work Rules" listed in the Employment Agreement. If you terminate an employee because of a rule violation, you should tell her the reason — *if you can prove it.* Never accuse an employee of something you cannot prove.

The Dismissal Process

It's never easy to find the words to tell an employee that you no longer desire her services. If you feel uncomfortable dismissing the home caregiver by yourself, have a neighbor, friend or relative in the room with you. (An alternate plan is to give the caregiver notice of her dismissal over the telephone.)

Here are examples of some of the things that you might wish to say when it comes to this plan of last resort:

"I'm sorry, but I don't feel that things are working out. I need someone who, (is stronger, can drive, can work more flexible hours, lives closer, has more experience, etc). Thank you for your time and help."

"You're falling down on the job. You arrive between a half hour and an hour late and you have missed several days work without notice; I need someone more dependable. I am sorry, but I have to give you notice of termination."

When you terminate an employee's services, make sure that you get back all keys she might have. Keep accurate documentation of the event and your reasons for termination.

This will protect you in case of later dispute. It is prudent to keep all records on all employees for future reference.

If the reason for dismissal is based on changes in your family's needs or circumstances, and you have been pleased with your caregiver's job performance, then you may want to give some type of bonus or severance pay, and if possible advance notice to allow her to find other work. You should also write a letter of recommendation under these conditions.

Criminal Actions

Possible criminal activity on the part of a home worker, of course, is another matter altogether. In this case, the best defense is a good offense. If you have selected your caregiver carefully, following the screening, interviewing and background checking suggestions in Chapters Five and Six, you aren't likely to have a serious problem of this nature. Nevertheless, it can happen in the best of families.

Each of the following criminal offenses is grounds for dismissal of your employee. Whether you elect to file criminal charges will depend upon several factors: Is the evidence clear enough to prevail in court? Do local law enforcement and courts treat such cases seriously or tend to favor the victim? Do you want to help protect others from this caregiver, or just to be rid of her? Are you willing to invest the time and energy required to support prosecution by the District Attorney?

These are difficult questions, some of which have more to do with one's view of civic responsibility than of the process of caring for your elder relative/friend. Consider your own goals and values and proceed according to the dictates of your heart.

That said, let's take a brief look at *theft, elder abuse*, and *substance abuse* by a home caregiver.

Theft

Caution and common sense are your best protections against loss of property. Don't tempt human nature: keep valuables out of reach, preferably out of sight. As a further precaution, you may wish to consider some or all of the following steps:

- Provide the caregiver a vehicle key only if driving the vehicle is part of the job
- Make parts of the house off limits; keep them locked.
- Do not give the caregiver access to the elder's checkbook or credit cards
- Provide only enough cash as needed for daily expenses
- Prevent access to medicine and liquor cabinets.

Here are some other suggestions for protecting yourself and your relative from theft and other criminal behavior:

- Secure all valuables, including jewelry, in a safe deposit box.
- Do not give wages in advance.
- Ask a friend or relative to drop in unannounced occasionally during the helper's work hours.
- Make certain that paychecks are filled out carefully so that changes to the dollar amount cannot be made.
- Be cautious in all money management matters.
- Contact the police if a serious offense is committed.

Should you become aware that an item is missing, first conduct a very complete search. After an unsuccessful search for missing items or money, notify the authorities promptly. Never hesitate to file a police report on missing items, even if you believe that employee theft can't be proved. Get a copy of the report. A properly filed police report is generally required for insurance purposes.

Note: Be certain never to accuse a home caregiver directly in cases of suspected theft. False accusations can lead to legal action against you. Let the police conduct the investigation and the court make the determination of guilt or innocence.

Elder Abuse

Like a seasoned professional, you must be alert and attuned to this danger throughout the home care experience. When discussing "how things are going" with the elder, listen closely for any hint of rough or indifferent physical care, or of threats that may have been made or any other intimidating behaviors.

Because some elders can be coerced into keeping quiet in abusive situations through fear of retaliation, you must also scan for the *unspoken* signs and symptoms of elder abuse. Such signs include eating too much or too little, insomnia or sleeping a great deal, withdrawal or depression, or, with confused elders, rocking or agitation.

Elder abuse is a crime which must not be tolerated. If you suspect it, contact your local Adult Protective Services office for advice. If you have proof, dismiss the employee immediately and contact the police.

Substance Abuse

After your worker is hired, certain signs may indicate a problem: the smell of liquor on her breath, slurred speech, unexplained bruises that she tries to hide, poor personal appearance and/or memory lapses.

What if you notice these signs? Please consult a professional who is familiar with substance abuse. At the least, ask a physician, psychologist, social worker or minister. Better, talk with a community agency which specializes in substance abuse. They will give you advice about how to speak with the helper about seeking help. There are a variety of centers that specialize in the treatment of adult chemical dependency.

The home caregiver with a substance abuse problem should not be allowed to continue working, and should not be reappointed unless and until a qualified professional has certified that she has undergone successful treatment and is now free of any drug or alcohol problem. It is also crucial that she be monitored for continuing participation in a recovery program.

The Elder Refuses Home Help

There will be times when an older person does not want any assistance and refuses to cooperate with home caregivers, no matter what. It is very important for you to understand why. The following is a list of reasons why some elders have difficulty in accepting help from others:

- Accepting help seems an admission of dependency.
- Concern about the cost of the service.
- Desire to have a family member, and not someone else, provide care.
- Fear of strangers in the house.
- Conflicting cultural backgrounds.
- Language barriers.

Once you understand why the elder is refusing assistance, you can begin to develop strategies to encourage her to accept help. Everyone wants to feel able to take care of themselves and to control their own destinies. The introduction of a stranger into the intimacy of a private home, at precisely the time an elder is feeling vulnerable, is never easy. Perhaps one way to help your relative deal with negative feelings is to focus on how accepting help in one area will help her function independently in other areas — and save money in the long run.

Keep in mind that, no matter how loving and kind a worker is, there may be times when the older person finds her unacceptable, perhaps for one or more of the reasons above. If this is the case with the older person in your life, you may not be able to do much more than encourage her to accept differences in people and insist that she allow the caregiver to do her job.

Of course, you could begin the hiring process all over again; but, as even a brief review of previous chapters would reveal, this is a labor-intensive process. The more pro-active solution lies in dealing with the elder's resistance before the home caregiver's first day on the job, or working to mediate small problems before they mushroom into large ones.

After the Employment Agreement is signed, give the new caregiver and the elder plenty of opportunity to get to know and feel comfortable with one another. Look for special feelings between the elder and caregiver, as well as any potential areas of friction or misunderstanding. Watch to see how comfortable the elder is with the home caregiver's presence. Spend time later on talking this over with the older person in private.

If, however, in spite of your best efforts, the elder is unhappy with the home care situation, it's okay to try other alternatives. If you've saved your telephone screening and job application forms, you can simply backtrack and try another worker. You may need to repeat certain time-consuming steps, but your patience and efforts will eventually pay off.

Notice of Unsatisfactory Performance

Date:

TO:_____
    Employee

_____
    Address

Dear

Please accept this as a written confirmation of our meeting reviewing your performance in your present position. As it was explained to you, your performance is unsatisfactory and requires substantial immediate improvement in the following ways:

I sincerely hope that you will make this improvement. We would like to retain you as a valued employee for our family.

Very truly,

cc: File

ELDER INFORMATION FORM

Name_____

Address_____

City/State/Zip_____

Telephone_____

Social Security Number_____

Medicare Number_____

Health Plan/Insurance ID_____

Veteran's Serial Number_____

Blood Type_____

Allergies_____

Family Member's Information:

Name_____

Address_____

City/State/Zip_____

Home Phone_____Work Phone_____

Employer_____Work Hours_____

Additional Family Member's Information:

Name_____

Address_____

City/State/Zip_____

Home Phone_____Work Phone_____

Employer_____Work Hours_____

Name_____

Address_____

City/State/Zip_____

Home Phone_____Work Phone_____

Employer_____Work Hours_____

Name_____

Address_____

City/State/Zip_____

Home Phone_____Work Phone_____

Employer_____Work Hours_____

Name_____

Address_____

City/State/Zip_____

Home Phone_____Work Phone_____

Employer_____Work Hours_____

EMERGENCY TELEPHONE NUMBERS

(Leave several emergency telephone numbers with your home caregiver. In addition to the names of several family members, it is also important to leave numbers for a close friend, a relative, and your family physician. Include the phone numbers for your local police, fire, ambulance services, and your poison information center. Other inclusions are listed on the Elder Information Form.)

DIAL _____**for police, fire or medical emergencies**
(911 in most localities; check phone directory for local number)

The address of this house is_____

Major cross streets are_____

The phone number is_____

Ambulance_____ Police_____ Fire_____

Pharmacy_____Poison Control_____

Doctor_____ at (   )_____

Doctor_____ at (   )_____

Spouse_____ at (   )_____

Family at home_____ at (   )_____

Family at work_____ at (   )_____

Family at work_____ at (   )_____

Neighbor_____ at (   )_____

Neighbor_____ at (   )_____

Friend_____ at (   )_____

Friend_____ at (   )_____

Friend_____ at (   )_____

Clergy_____ at (   )_____

Chapter Nine

FINDING AND USING COMMUNITY RESOURCES

"Emma has been an inspiration to me. Although she is mentally impaired, she could easily teach a lot of us how to live life. As I went about my chores in caring for her, she would take me by the arm and ask, 'Shall we whistle or shall we sing?' I often think of Emma when times are hard. I say to myself, 'Well, shall we whistle or shall we sing?' "
— Judith Ellen Brooks, Home Helper

YOU AND I LIVE IN THE REAL WORLD. OUR BEST-LAID PLANS and schedules seldom fall neatly into place.

As convenient as it might be to employ a home caregiver to provide for the needs of your aging loved one, chances are it will be more complicated than that. Your real-world plan will likely include a mix of available caregivers and services:

- You
- Family members
- Employed home caregiver
- Friends
- Neighbors
- Neighborhood and community resources
- Professional services and facilities.

This chapter will help you sort out who does what, when and how.

As you piece together the eldercare puzzle, begin by honestly figuring out how much care you yourself are personally willing and able to provide. It's virtually impossible to do it all yourself because of the competing demands of your own work and family.

Look closely at the gaps that remain in your care plan and calendar, and start filling them with a creative patchwork of family resources. A variety of family members (spouse, siblings, young adults, in-laws) may be willing to help out with home care tasks.

Where to from there? Turn outward to your neighborhood and community. Friends, neighbors, shopkeepers, utility personnel, clergy and others can also help.

Community resources for caregiving are amazingly plentiful. Headquartered in or near one's neighborhood or community, they are close-at-hand and convenient, and may be informally connected in some sort of care "network." These local services tend to be less medically-oriented, and usually include adult day care, home-delivered meals, respite care and hospice care.

Other examples center around "residential alternatives" — care settings for frail elders that fall somewhere between home and nursing home in terms of the level of care provided. Some examples of residential alternatives to nursing homes include assisted living facilities and continuing care retirement communities.

The examples mentioned here represent only a tiny sampling of the full range of community services. The scope of this book does not permit a complete discussion, and readers are urged to learn more on their own. Good places to start include Area Agencies on Aging, hospital-based senior care programs and geriatric care managers. Several progressive corporations and businesses are now also beginning to provide eldercare consultation and referral assistance as an employee benefit.

As mentioned throughout the book, constructing a workable plan for long term care is perhaps the greatest challenge in consumer-directed eldercare. No book can tell you exactly how to do this, as each family's situation is unique. General guidelines do apply, however, and this includes the caveat to seek *multiple sources* of assistance.

A Family Conference

A family meeting or conference is a good way to launch a cooperative effort for care of a family elder. As a forum for sharing information and feelings, it can improve communication and cooperation among family members.

Be very clear about the purpose of the family meeting, and about the topics to be discussed. Jot down the kinds of help that will be needed. Have a list of tasks that can be assumed in as much detail as possible.

As a rough agenda for your family meeting, consider the topics covered in this book:

- How much and what kind of care does our elder need?
- How is each family member able to contribute to care?
- What community agencies are available for help?
- Do we want to hire a caregiver?
- If so, what tasks will we assign to her?
- How many hours a week do we need her?
- Will we need to hire backup help also, or can family members cover?
- Who will: Do the recruiting? Handle the background checks? Make the hiring decision? Supervise her work? Write the paychecks? Handle the taxes? Buy

needed insurance coverage? Submit insured
expenses for payment?
- Should we consider a home care agency?
- Is skilled nursing or other health care required?
- Who will maintain contact with the physician and
  other health care providers?

You'll want to personalize the agenda to fit your own family
situation.

Don't expect things to go smoothly. These conferences have
a way of heating up long-simmering family issues to the
boiling point. The result can be hurt feelings, and even
estrangement, which is the last thing you want when you are
trying to clear the home care hurdles.

Having a social worker or a member of the clergy present
for your family meeting can be helpful. The steadying presence
of one of these professionals can help families successfully and
creatively find solutions to the most challenging dilemmas
surrounding an elder's care.

Sharing the Caring at Home

Each family member brings a different set of contributions
to the challenge of home care. Some may offer financial
assistance; others, the administrative functions of setting up
appointments and coordinating services; still others, hands-on
personal care of the older person. But, even when the family's
resources are maximized by creative planning, and then
reinforced with additional help from friends and neighbors,
the care plan may fall short of the elder's needs. Then it's time
to look outside of the family and its extended network to
community services.

This chapter provides a simplified "road map" to help you
chart your course through the maze of home and
community-based services. But in spite of your background
reading, you'll find yourself making false starts and detours,

hesitating at crossroads, and almost certainly running up against the occasional dead end. In that event, this chapter may provide enough information to sharpen your resolve to continue the journey. Remember, help is available to those resourceful and persistent enough to seek it out.

Community-based services for elders can be found in almost any social service setting. They are offered by public, private, commercial, nonprofit, civic, fraternal and religious organizations. Perhaps the best place to begin is with Area Agencies on Aging.

Area Agencies on Aging

Often called "Triple A's," these nonprofit outfits play a central role in helping elders manage at home and in their communities. AAAs don't provide many direct services; their job is largely to plan, fund and monitor the vast network of programs provided for under the Older Americans Act. Details about the in-home, transportation, legal and social services provided through AAAs can be found in Appendix D.

There are over 670 Area Agencies on Aging across the United States. Through its "provider" agencies, each AAA has the responsibility for information and referral, home-based supportive services, nutrition and other programs. The entire system is overseen by the Administration on Aging, a part of the U.S. Department of Health and Human Services.

Older Americans Act services are not income-based. That is, anyone age 60-plus is eligible. Of course, as with most governmental programs, service priorities are set according to greatest social and economic need.

As Area Agencies go by a variety of names, their numbers are sometimes difficult to find in the telephone directory. If you have trouble, the best bet for finding the telephone number for the AAA in your area is to call the Eldercare Locator Service, listed in Appendix C. You might also contact your State Unit on Aging (SUA).

SUAs are the focal point in each state for activities on behalf of older citizens. SUAs plan and coordinate the provision of social and personal care services, and provide leadership and guidance to the AAAs. SUAs and AAAs are part of the multi-level administrative structure established by the Older Americans Act of 1965, often referred to as the "Aging Network." Funds flow from Congress, through the Administration on Aging in Washington, through the Aging Network, and ultimately to local communities where they provide a multitude of services. A listing of SUAs can be found in Appendix F.

(Editor's Note: Once again, it is appropriate to note that there is currently much political discussion about cutting back on federally sponsored social programs. Aging services may be vulnerable under a widespread cost-and-services-reduction effort. It is hoped that AAAs and SUAs will survive any such cutbacks, but nothing is assured.)

Adult Day Care

Adult day care centers are designed to care for frail elders who should not be left alone during the day. Quiet games, sing-alongs, dancing and physical exercise offer pleasant and stimulating outlets for frail or confused elders.

Typically, families use adult day care four to eight hours per day, one to five days per week. (In some settings, adult day care is offered on weekends, although this is not as common.) A hot noon meal, and sometimes transportation to and from the center, are typically provided.

Adult day care services are operated by hospitals, nursing homes, religious organizations, proprietary organizations and Area Agencies on Aging. They are either free or on a donation or fee-for-service basis. Most insurances do not reimburse for adult day care.

Day care centers are staffed by trained, salaried nurses, social workers and aides, as well as by volunteers. Some medically-oriented centers provide medical care, physical therapy and rehabilitation. (Reimbursement through Medicaid applies to some medically-oriented centers.)

Home-delivered Meals

When an elder is incapacitated to the point that it is difficult for her to get to the grocery store or prepare a meal, home-delivered meals can be a lifesaver.

Often termed "meals-on-wheels," these nutrition programs are a certerpiece of the services funded by the Older Americans Act and administered in local communities by the AAAs. (Proprietary for-profit agencies are also involved in providing home-delivered meals on a fee-for-service basis in many communities.) A hot, nutritious meal is delivered to the doorstep of those who qualify. Donations are accepted from those who are able and willing to contribute. As there is often a waiting list for this desirable service, those who are recuperating after a hospital stay or suffering from very debilitating chronic illnesses are often given highest priority.

Respite Care

Respite is temporary care designed to provide relief to family members or others who need a break from the strains of caregiving. Relief may be given at home, or in a nursing home or assisted living setting. Family caregivers generally place "respite" services at the very top of their list as a most desirable service option.

In-home respite allows caregivers to get out of the house for a short while — to run errands, attend religious services, visit with friends, or whatever it takes to renew themselves physically and emotionally. A homemaker, aide or companion temporarily takes over care of the elder, to cook and clean, to bathe and groom, or simply to provide companionship. To learn more about respite care, call your Area Agency on Aging.

Facility-based respite provides caregiver relief for varying periods of time: overnight, for a few days, or during a family vacation. In a hospital nursing home or other supervised residential setting, trained staff provide direct supportive care to the elder on a 24-hour-a-day basis.

Respite care, while sometimes available at no charge through nonprofit or voluntary agencies, is most often purchased by the caregiver from home care agencies. Respite fees generally are not reimbursable through insurances. Fees average about $10 an hour at this writing.

Family-to-family respite: In some communities no formally organized respite services exist. But the need for respite is still there, no matter how small the community, or how isolated the individual family may be. In such a situation, one of the simplest yet most effective ways of providing respite care is "neighbors helping neighbors" or, one family sharing caregiving tasks with another, then trading off so that each family gets respite in turn. Even a single hour of relief can make all the difference.

Hospice Care

Hospices are certified and licensed organizations that provide skilled nursing care to those who are gravely ill; that is, individuals expected to live no longer than six months. Comfort, relief from pain and death with dignity are central tenets.

If you elect hospice care, a team of workers — usually a doctor, nurse, social worker, home health aide, clergy and volunteers — will help the terminally ill elder make the most of the time remaining. The team also provides respite care, home caregiver services and bereavement counseling for family members.

Hospice care is usually available 24 hours a day, seven days a week, in either a home or in a long-term care facility. When hospice is delivered at home, it incorporates many of the consumer-directed values discussed in this book.

Local hospitals, social services departments, Visiting Nurse Associations, disease-related associations and religious organizations can refer you to hospice services. Medicare-certified hospice care costs are covered if the illness is determined to be terminal by a physician.

COMMUNITY SERVICES FOR FRAIL ELDERS

Adult Day Care
What: supervision and services for frail or confused older people
Where: nursing home, senior center, social service agency, private for-profit adult day care centers, personal care homes
Payment: sliding scale, donation, third party or fee

Respite Care
What: temporary relief from caregiving
Where: in-home, nursing home, hospital or assisted-living facility, personal care homes
Payment: free, sliding scale, or fee

Home-delivered Meals
What: hot meal delivered to the home
Where: in-home
Payment: donation or fee for service

Hospice Care
What: support for the terminally ill and their families
Where: hospital or community agency
Payment: third-party or fee

Relocation

Nine-out-of-ten elders express a strong preference for living out their lives at home. Most of us are unwilling to move out of our homes without extremely compelling reasons. This surely has to do with home's comfort, privacy and familiarity, coupled with its links to precious family memories. Certainly, when it comes to living longer and living better, home is best most of the time.

The day may come, however, when you realize that consumer-directed home care is not working out, even with the assistance of family members, friends, a reliable home caregiver, and other formal and informal home- and community-based supports. It's important not to cling to independence beyond the point of reasonableness. Relocation to a more supportive setting is at times the better part of wisdom, and can be managed with style, dignity and satisfaction.

Supportive housing refers to a variety of living arrangements for persons who require some degree of assistance, from help with bathing and grooming, to help with medical care. Based upon the condition of the elder's health, relocation options might include the following:

Assisted Living Facilities. Elders who need only a little extra help or general supervision are often likely candidates for an assisted living arrangement. Meals are shared and housekeeping is provided. Transportation and social and recreational activities are often included in the total package. The atmosphere is "familylike."

Assisted living facilities range in size from single family homes for one or two older persons, to large facilities serving, in some cases, hundreds of residents. They are usually licensed by the state to provide a basic level of care. These residential settings may be referred to by many names, including *domiciliary care homes, adult foster care homes, personal care homes, sheltered housing,* and, more recently, *board and care homes.*

While costs are lower than nursing homes, almost all assisted living residents pay privately. In other words, insurance doesn't reimburse for the costs associated with assisted living. Many residents do use Social Securit and special state supplements to help pay for assisted living.

Continuing Care Retirement Communities (CCRCs). CCRCs typically combine a large, sprawling campus with a full complement of services and a variety of personal and health care options. Such facilities offer the comfort of knowing that as needs change, services will be available on-site. This is because independent units, assisted living units and medical care facilities are typically all housed together on the same CCRC campus.

CCRC residents are entitled to a living unit, meals, housekeeping, transportation and activities. Additionally, health care services — up to skilled nursing home care — may be covered completely or in part, depending on the community selected.

Most individuals enter the CCRC at the independent level, often with the option of having some meals provided; and move, as needed, through the various levels of care.

CCRCs tend to be one of the more expensive supportive housing options. A sizable "down payment" in the form of an endowment is often charged, in addition to monthly fees. CCRCs often appeal to upper-income elders, who, having weighed their financial options, opt for CCRCs as a kind of long-term care insurance.

Nursing Homes. There comes a time for many elders and families when nursing homes must be given serious consideration. In many cases, placement in a nursing home is a positive step. Nursing home staff can cope with such things as frequent falling, incontinence, poor nutrition, infection and behavioral problems. Twenty-four-hour medical care is provided for those who have a disabling chronic condition. Nursing homes are also used for short-term rehabilitation after discharge from a hospital. Pre-admission screening will probably be required prior to admission to any nursing home to determine the appropriate level of care. Costs (1995) typically range from $2,500 to $3,500 per month ($30,000 to $42,000 a year) for skilled nursing care, room and board. That doesn't include the cost of medication. Medicaid may help pay for the cost of nursing home care for those who have income and assets at near national poverty levels.

Why would your family choose any of these supportive housing alternatives? You could decide that access to 24-hour staff and health status monitoring adds peace of mind. Or that, without family or friends nearby, supportive housing would be a better option for providing the elder with a welcome sense of community and companionship.

Finding and Paying for Supportive Housing

To find out more about the kinds, locations and prices of the various kinds of supportive housing available to elders, call the local Area Agency on Aging. AAAs sometimes maintain a registry of housing facilities from which they make referrals, or, some AAAs have developed listings which may be mailed out to you. If the AAA does not maintain a housing registry, they should be able to refer you to an organization that does. Or, ask the AAA for the number of the state licensure agency responsible for the regulation of supportive housing for older citizens. (If you have difficulty locating your AAA, the Information operator may be able to help you locate the licensure agency.)

Licensure agencies are charged with assuring that facilities with the "supportive housing" designation are indeed that, rather than merely rooming houses. In Florida, the Agency for

Health Care Administration maintains a file of inspection reports, open to public review, listing any recent citations issued by state inspection teams.

If you are searching for a suitable nursing home, call your regional Long Term Care Ombudsman Program. They may be willing to provide a listing of the nursing homes in your area, or they may have files listing problems with certain long-term care facilities.

Some states fund health councils that are charged in part with educating the public on the availability of health and rehabilitative facilities. These councils sometimes produce publications that compare and contrast the amenities of various types of supportive housing, to assist you in making the best choice.

Nursing homes are one of the few supportive housing alternatives that are potentially reimbursable by Medicare, Medicaid and private insurers. Keep in mind that the reimbursement picture is shifting constantly, but at this writing (1995), most people pay for supportive housing directly out of their life savings or personal income.

The housing market for elders is extremely complex and constantly developing. While only a thumb-nail sketch of senior housing is provided here, those who wish to delve more deeply into housing options will find helpful resources in their local bookstore.

* * * * * *

Entering the world of home- and community-based services for elders can be like finding yourself in a huge, bustling airport in a foreign country. You don't speak the language, there are a hundred gates to choose from, make one wrong move and you'll miss your plane! It may be hard to believe things could be so extraordinarily complex and confusing, but they truly are.

This chapter gave you an overview of services that are widely available in many parts of the country. You may discover other services that are unique to your locale.

One way to familiarize yourself with this new terrain is to hire a guide: a geriatric care manager or other knowledgeable professional. If this is a luxury that you can't afford, or if you simply prefer to find your way independently, begin by contacting the Area Agency on Aging. AAAs hold the key to the world of aging services, and can set you on the path of successful exploration on your own.

Chapter Ten

DEALING WITH TAXES, INSURANCE, AND LAWS

"Paying taxes the old way was very annoying, and a lot of damn trouble. You had to take the net amount, apply a certain percentage for the Social Security part and the Medicare part, then add the two together. I've gotten to where I'm not much of a bookkeeper anymore, so I'm glad for a new system of reporting."

— Mike Hinson, age 80, Household Employer

F OR SOME PEOPLE, AVOIDING PAPERWORK IS REASON ENOUGH to hire through an agency. Others find the paperwork manageable, and appreciate the greater flexibility and control they gain by taking charge of their own payments and records.

This chapter will explain your tax and legal responsibilities as a household employer, outlining the requirements for withholding and paying taxes. It will also explain the forms you must give your employees, those your employees must give you, and those you must send to the Internal Revenue Service (IRS) and the Social Security Administration (SSA). Finally, you will be introduced to the issues of potential tax deductions, and other important topics, including employer's insurance, labor laws and the how-tos of employing immigrants.

This chapter will give you a basic overview of what you're up against in each important category, however *this discussion is in no way intended to render legal, accounting or other professional advice. If legal advice or other expert assistance is required, the services of a competent professional person should be sought.*

What's an Employer To Do?

As the employer of a home caregiver, your basic responsibilities will include familiarity with:

- *Taxes*, including Tax Identification Numbers, federal income tax withholding, Social Security taxes (FICA), Federal Unemployment Tax (FUTA), state taxes, self-employed worker ("independent contractor") rules, tax deductions and credits for dependent care, and employee record-keeping requirements.
- *Insurance*, including Worker's Compensation insurance, liability insurance, and bonding.
- *Labor Laws*, including federal and state wage and hour requirements and the regulations for immigrant workers.

Sound intimidating? It needn't be. The worst part will be reading through the government forms for the first time! Suggestion: use a yellow highlighter as you read, and call the SSA or IRS whenever you have questions. IRS can be reached by calling 1-800-829-1040; you may reach the Social Security Administration by calling 1-800-772-1213.

When you call one of these national 800 numbers, you will hear a recorded voice recite a lengthy "menu" of taped information options. The tapes cover the most typically-asked questions, but it's also important to know that you can talk to a real-live human being if you so desire. Staff are usually patient, knowledgeable and helpful.

You may also wish to access some of the sources of aid that may be available in your own community. For instance, the

U.S. Small Business Administration sponsors the Service Corps of Retired Executives (SCORE), which is a nonprofit association providing free business counseling. SCORE volunteers, who are retired and active business executives, offer one-on-one consultation on accounting, taxation and other aspects of business management.

Of course, another way to get started is to schedule and pay for a consultation with an accountant, but it may be easier than you think to take the do-it-yourself approach. Once you are "in the system," the IRS will automatically mail you the forms you need, providing reminders of when you should do what.

Keep in mind that tax laws are subject to frequent changes. As this is written — shortly after the 1994 U.S. national elections — many political analysts are predicting big changes in the next few years. No one can safely predict the political future, but one bit of advice will work in virtually all situations: *ask lots of questions and stay informed!* Ask your congressperson, the IRS, the SSA, your accountant, your librarian. Accurate, up-to- date information will be your best ally in the tax wars.

"Nanny Taxes"

Your tax-related responsibilities as an employer of in-home workers were greatly simplified October 22, 1994. On this date, "Nanny Tax" legislation — or, to use the more official terminology, "Employment Taxes for Household Employees" — was signed into law, making the payment of this type of employment tax relatively painless.

You'll recall that several national political figures, including a nominee for Attorney General of the United States, made national news in 1993 and 1994 for mishandling taxes for child-care workers. Largely as a result of that publicity, Congress decided that the arcane laws needed an overhaul.

Under the old system, quarterly reporting and payment of taxes was required for every employee who earned over $50 in a quarter. Now, the wage threshold has been raised to $1,000 a year, and reporting is only required once, rather than four times. Many of the IRS forms used under the old system have become obsolete (as of January 1, 1995). Now, instead of reporting on the old IRS Forms 942 and 940, you will do so on your federal income tax return.

(While the new law makes things easier for new employers, it complicates matters somewhat for those who employed household workers and paid quarterly taxes during 1994. Since the higher wage threshold was retroactive to January 1, 1994, household employers and employees who paid social security and Medicare taxes on 1994 wages of less than $1,000 during that year are eligible for refunds. Refunds with interest are available by filing Form 843.)

Questions regarding the technicalities of the Nanny Tax legislation should be directed to the Taxpayer Service Division of the IRS office nearest you. Get IRS Publication 926, *Employment Taxes for Household Employers*, for more information on the latest reporting requirements.

Your best bet for finding the correct address and telephone number of a local IRS office is probably in the "blue pages" of your local telephone directory or by calling Information.

Tax Identification Numbers

Employer Identification Number. Before you get started, it's important to note that all employers must have a federal Employer Identification Number (EIN). This is not the same as a Social Security number. If you hire or plan to hire a home caregiver but do not have an Employer Identification Number, apply for one by filing Form SS-4 (*Application for Employer Identification Number*). You can get this form at Social Security Administration offices, or by calling the toll-free IRS number 1-800-829-1040. Or you may apply for your EIN by telephone using the same number.

Employee's Social Security Number (SSN). Every employee must have a Social Security number. As an employer, you must obtain each employees' name and SSN, and enter them on the annual Form W-2, *Wage and Tax Statement*, which you must give to employees by January 31 each year. If you do not provide the correct name and SSN, you may owe a penalty. Any employee without a Social Security card can get one by completing Form SS-5, *Application for a Social Security Card*. You can get this form at Social Security Administration offices or by calling 1- 800-772-1213.

Federal Income Tax Withholding

You do not have to withhold income tax on wages paid to a home caregiver unless she asks for it and you agree. If this is the case, the employee must give you a completed IRS Form W-4 (available at IRS offices and many Post Offices.) You must withhold an amount from each wage payment based on the Form W-4 and the tax tables in Circular E, *Employer's Tax Guide*.

Social Security Taxes

One of your main tax-paying responsibilities as a household employer will be paying social security and Medicare taxes. (These taxes are referred to as FICA taxes — shorthand for the Federal Insurance Compensation Act.) You must withhold the employee's share of taxes each time you pay wages, and you must pay an equal amount from your own funds once a year when you pay your federal income tax. (You may pay the home caregiver's share of Social Security taxes if you want to, as a form of additional compensation to the caregiver. In this case, no deductions are made from paychecks. You, the employer, pay the total amount of taxes due at the end of the year.)

The FICA tax rate changes periodically. Contact your Social Security office to get the most current rate. For example, the tax rate for 1995 for both the employer and the employee is 7.65

percent each. This means that, each time you write a check to your home caregiver for her wages, you should deduct and withhold 7.65 percent of the total amount paid. At the end of the year, when you file your return, you will match these amounts with your own contribution of 7.65 percent of her salary. Thus, the total Social Security tax on each wage payment is 15.3 percent.

Example: On January 19, 1995, Carmela Martini hires Delores Painchaud to provide housekeeping and personal care services for her 90-year-old mother. Delores works three days a week, earning $150 a week. Because Mrs. Martini pays Delores more than $1,000 in cash wages for the year ($150 a week x 52 weeks = $7,800), she must withhold a total of 7.65% from each of Delores' weekly paychecks to cover FICA taxes. This amounts to $11.48 per week ($150 x .0765). At the end of the year, Mrs. Martini will report and pay to the IRS the total amount she withheld from Ms. Painchaud's paychecks, and will match this sum with an equal amount from her own pocket. In other words, for every $11.48 withheld from Delores' paycheck, another $11.48 will be paid by Mrs. Martini at the end of the year to cover FICA taxes.

Note: Beginning in 1995, household employment wages paid to workers under age 18 are exempt from Social Security and Medicare taxes unless household employment is the worker's principal occupation.

Federal Unemployment Tax

The Federal Unemployment Tax Act (FUTA), with state unemployment systems, provides for payments of unemployment compensation to workers who have lost their jobs. Most employers pay both federal and state unemployment tax. Only the employer pays this tax; it is not deducted from the employee's wages. As of January 1, 1995, household employers will no longer use Forms 940 or 940-EZ,

Employer's Annual Federal Unemployment (FUTA) Tax Return, to report Federal unemployment tax. This tax will be reported and paid once a year on the employer's own federal income tax return if $1,000 or more in wages has been paid per quarter.

Beginning in 1995, household employers are not required to make a quarterly deposit of this tax, as sometimes was the case under the old system. You'll pay Uncle Sam once a year, using the forms mentioned above.

(Isn't this fun?)

State Taxes

You can find out what your state does in relation to employment taxes by calling your state's department of labor or department of employment. You may, for example, need to withhold a percentage of earnings for state unemployment taxes.

States have their own specific regulations regarding wages paid, so it's up to you to determine your responsibilities as an employer in your particular state. For instance, many states require employers to pay a higher minimum wage than does the federal law. Some require payment of overtime wages — usually at a higher rate — for hours worked in excess of eight in a day. State laws and regulations also vary greatly with regard to how often employees have to be paid, and how soon after termination. Your employee must be paid according to the law in your state, and it's your responsibility to know those requirements.

Self-employed Workers: The "Independent Contractor"

Families who need paid caregivers sometimes attempt to get around tax responsibilities by using *independent contractors* rather than employees. In an independent contractor arrangement, the worker uses her own equipment, sets her own hours, supervises herself, and may work for several employers. An independent contractor is responsible for filing her own Social Security and Medicare payments, and reporting her income as a self-employed worker. She is also responsible for purchasing her own worker's compensation or other insurance coverages.

Sound appealing? Before you get excited, you should know that it's not easy for a worker to qualify. Look carefully before jumping into an independent contractor arrangement. The IRS has *very* stringent qualifications for independent contractors — essentially taking a "guilty until proven innocent" view: they consider your worker to be an employee unless you can prove she's an independent contractor.

For your further guidance, here's the IRS language:

"Anyone who performs services is an employee if you, as an employer, can control what will be done and how it will be done. This is so even when you give the employee freedom of action. What matters is that you have the legal right to control the method and result of the services."

Should the IRS ever question your use of self-employed workers as a possible tax-dodging ploy, the burden of proof — and any penalties — will fall upon you, not the worker.

If you and your caregiver get into a dispute at some future time, your arrangement may be questioned. Some elders and families have been sued for back wages by disgruntled former workers, often resulting in reports to state wage-and-hour boards, the IRS and other regulatory bodies.

Protect yourself before you hire a caregiver by getting up-to-date information on tax laws and wage-and-hour laws from the IRS, state tax board, and state regulatory agencies. Use a written agreement which makes clear whether the arrangement is for an employee or an independent contractor. Keep accurate records of hours worked and amounts paid and file receipts or cancelled checks.

For more information on independent contractors, call the IRS at 1-800-829-1040 and ask for Publication 937: *Employment Taxes*, or call your Social Security office and ask for a free copy of *If You're Self-Employed* (Publication No. 05-10022).

If you want IRS to decide your worker's status for you, you may file Form SS-8, *Determination of Employee Work Status for Purposes of Federal Employment Taxes and Income Tax Withholding,* available at IRS offices.

SCHEDULE OF TAX RESPONSIBILITIES FOR HOUSEHOLD EMPLOYERS

WHAT	WHEN	FORM
Pay at least $4.25 per hour to home caregiver	**At time of hire**	**N/A**
Check to make sure of caregiver's U.S. citizenship or legal authorization to work in the U.S.	**At time of hire**	**NS Form I-9**
Have each home caregiver complete a status form for withholding federal income tax	**At time of hire and annually**	**W-4**
Pay employment taxes one time each year for each home caregiver	**4/15 for previous year**	**Federal income return 1040**
Pay any applicable state taxes	**As per state law**	**Tax office**
Provide each employee with a wage and tax statement	**January 31 for previous year**	**IRS Forms W-2**

Mail a copy of the Form W-2 to Social Security Administration's Wilkes-Barre (PA) Center.

Tax Deductions And Credits For Caregiving

Deductions for Health Care Services: When it comes to deducting the costs of home help for tax purposes, it depends on what kind of work is done. The secret of deductibility lies in convincing IRS that home caregivers are providing the equivalent of nursing care. If the services are not clearly medical in nature, you can expect questions from the IRS. By all accounts, the outcome can go either way. A number of taxpayers report success in audits or appeals in personal care cases.

Precedent has shown that home caregiver duties have been ruled as "nursing-like" services and are deductible; but remember, the usual housekeeping chores and cleaning are not. It is best to get a statement from your doctor which includes:

- A description of the medical condition, whether it is permanent, and the cause and date of its onset.
- A complete list of the help needed.
- A statement of whether you need live-in or daily help.

These are only general guidelines. It is best to contact the IRS office in Washington, D.C. at 1-800-829-1040. Explain what you are paying, and request a letter from them stating what you are allowed as a deduction. The use of personal care workers comes under the section on *Tax Laws of Special Interest.* Regulations for this code are available at district offices of the IRS. Once you get a letter from the IRS stating what is allowable, file a copy of it every year with your tax return. It should help minimize the problem of additional audits.

Dependent Care Tax Credit: If you are the working caregiver of a dependent elder, and the two of you live together in the same household, you may be entitled to the "dependent care credit" when paying Federal income tax. For instance, if, due to physical or mental incapacity, the elder needs help with grooming, eating or getting to the bathroom, and you must hire a home helper so you can go to work, you qualify.

This tax advantage is especially intriguing because it allows for the deduction of non-medical expenses. For instance, if your home caregiver does housekeeping, cooking and personal care services, partly for the benefit of the elder, the entire expense can be included. It is possible that the taxpayer can deduct, directly from the tax owed for the year — as much as $720 for one qualifying dependent, and up to $1,440 if there are two or more dependents receiving care. Remember, this is a credit against your taxes rather than a deduction from your gross income. Also, this credit is phased out as a taxpayer's adjusted gross income increases.

See the IRS Publication No. 503, *Child and Dependent Care Expenses*, for more instructions. You can order this and other IRS publications by calling 1-800-TAX-FORM (1-800-829-3676). You can also write to the IRS Forms Distribution Center nearest you. Check your income tax package for the address.

And, once again, remember that the laws do change! Tax credits may not always be available; check frequently to stay up to date.

Dependent Care Assistance Programs: Some employers offer Dependent Care Assistance Programs (DCAPs) to help their employees pay for home care expenses. The name of the benefit program may vary from employer to employer, but the principle is the same — you redirect part of your salary to a special account that is used exclusively for the care of an elder. This applies in cases where the elder spends eight hours a day in your home, and is physically or mentally incapable of self-care. The money put into this account is not subject to federal income tax, Social Security tax, or state income tax. The exceptions are Pennsylvania and New Jersey where DCAPs are subject to state taxes.

A DCAP is an opportunity to save money on your dependent care expenses; however, you should investigate a DCAP arrangement thoroughly before committing money. DCAPs can be complicated until you have experience with them. Discuss your particular situation with your employer's Employee Assistance Program (EAP) or benefits office and with your professional tax advisor.

Employee Records

You must keep tax-related records for at least 4 years. These should be available for IRS review. Your records should contain:

- Your employer identification number,
- Copies of tax returns you have filed,
- Dates and amounts of all wage payments you have made,
- Copies of each employee's tax withholding allowance certificate (Form W-4),
- Any employee copies of Form W-2 that were returned to you as undeliverable.

It is important to have a file card on each home caregiver, even those who may have been employed for only weeks or days. Include the name, address, phone number, date of birth, social security number, driver's license number, date hired and date left employment. The name on the file card should be recorded exactly as it appears on the home caregiver's social security card. If the name shown on the social security card is different from the name the home caregiver uses, including name changes due to marriage or divorce, tell her to contact the Social Security office and get a new card that reflects her current name.

(If your home caregiver does not have a Social Security number, you should require that she apply for one. See page 143.)

Also, keep copies of all formal written documents and communications, from the application form, to background check records, to performance ratings. It's also helpful to keep a copy of your original job advertisement and all your notes pertaining to the job interview. Documentation is the key to protecting yourself in the unlikely event that you are charged with violating an employee's legal rights.

Insurance Policies

Worker's Compensation Insurance. Worker's Compensation insurance — which pays the worker for medical expenses and lost income resulting from an injury on the job — historically has not been required for home workers. Recently, however, many states have begun to include household workers under their worker's compensation laws.

Ask your insurance broker, the state insurance commission, or the worker's compensation agency in your state about worker's compensation for domestic employees, and find out if your employee should be covered under this system.

Keep in mind that this coverage benefits the worker, not the employer.

Liability Insurance. If your worker slips and falls and hurts her back or otherwise injures herself, or if she is injured by the elder, or if she damages property or causes personal injury, you may have big problems. It is wise to protect your family by maximizing the comprehensive liability portion of your homeowner's insurance policy. Make sure that it includes coverage for in-home employees injured on the job. Phone the insurance agent who services your homeowner's policy and see if you can attach a rider to cover household employees.

If your present homeowner's policy is not adequate, even with a rider, you will probably need a separate policy. It is highly desirable to provide for such protection since you face the potential liability for the costs and damages of a lawsuit when these coverages are not maintained. So-called "umbrella liability" coverage is sold in million-dollar units at quite modest premiums (under $150 at this writing for the first million dollars of coverage).

Bonding. Although bonding is one form of protection for an employer, it does not insure that the worker is qualified to provide safe and satisfactory care. It means only that the home caregiver carries an insurance policy that protects her from claims filed against her. If you sued a bonded home helper, for instance, because you believed that she stole money or property, the bond would cover the loss. That is, if you won the case by proving in a court of law that the employee stole the items, and the court awarded you a settlement, the bonding company would pay. Of course, bonding covers only proven theft.

Bonds can be obtained for individuals by paying a fixed dollar amount. If an incident occurred and the court ruled the employee guilty, you should be able to collect the value of the property stolen from the bonding company, provided the value does not exceed the amount of the bond. For example, if a $10,000 ring is stolen, but the employee was bonded for only $5,000, then $5,000 would be all that you could recover.

The cost of a bond varies depending on the amount of the bond and number of employees to be covered. The smallest premium typically will be about $100, which at this writing in Florida purchases about $10,000 worth of insurance for a year.

To purchase this kind of insurance, contact a local insurance agency and request information on the purchase of a "business services bond." You might start close to home by asking your own family insurance agency. Many times, the same companies that sell life insurance and auto insurance also sell business services bonds. If your insurance carrier does not offer this product, a "surety company" will. Preferred National Insurance and Old Republic Surety Company are two large national concerns. Or, simply check the Yellow Pages under "Bonds - Surety and Fidelity."

Once you have identified a vendor, the bond may usually be purchased over the telephone. The home caregiver should make the call herself, because the bond will be issued in her name. A clerk will ask questions and fill out an application; the information gathered will pertain exclusively to the home caregiver's own situation and personal financial status.

Even though the bond will be purchased by the employee in her name, elders and families should consider reimbursing her for the cost of the bond. While the protection offered by bonding in home care situations is slim, it is usually the family which has the most to lose in terms of money and property, and therefore the most to gain from the purchase of a surety bond.

Labor Laws

It would be foolhardy to launch into the employment enterprise without having a passing knowledge of both federal and state labor laws that protect the rights of all workers, including household workers. You don't have to be an attorney, but to proceed in ignorance, or to just ignore these laws, could certainly lead to problems down the road. Fortunately, the laws that apply to employers of less than twenty workers — which will include virtually all families and elders employing home caregivers — are not difficult to understand. They mostly relate to minimum wage, overtime, equal pay, employment of minors, and employment of immigrant workers.

Minimum Wage. With a few exceptions, the Federal minimum wage of $4.25 per hour must be paid. (Some states require a higher minimum.)

Overtime Pay. Time-and-a-half (one and one-half times the regular rate of pay) must be paid to hourly employees for every hour worked over forty in a week or over eight in a day.

Equal Pay. Equal pay is due to men and women for substantially equal work done under similar circumstances.

Employment of Minors. Youths 16 and 17 may work at anytime for unlimited hours in home caregiving jobs; youths aged 14 and 15 may work outside of school hours; minors under the age of thirteen should not be employed.

For more detailed information regarding the Federal labor laws summarized above, consult the nearest office of the Wage and Hour Division, which you can find in the phone book under U.S. Government, Department of Labor, Employment Standards Administration.

As mentioned previously in this chapter, many states have laws which vary from the federal standards, notably when it comes to the basics of wages and overtime payments. For more detailed information, contact the Wage and Hour Division of your state's employment department or labor department.

For an excellent review of the federal labor laws as they relate to home caregivers, request a free copy of *How the Fair Labor Standards Act Applies to Domestic Service Workers* from the U.S. Department of Labor, Employment Standards Administration, Wage and Hour Division (202-219-4907). Ask for *WP Publication 1382*, or, *WH Publication 1282, Handy Reference Guide to the Fair Labor Standards Act.* These publications are also usually available through regional offices of the U.S. Department of Labor.

Employment of Immigrant Workers. Immigrants represent a good source of home care personnel. But remember, if you hire *unauthorized* immigrant workers, you are liable for criminal prosecution and fines. Fortunately, employers can hire immigrants with out risking fines if they follow the simple steps outlined below.

For each new hire, you must verify that the home caregiver is authorized to work by completing a form known as the "I-9." U.S. Immigration and Naturalization Services (INS) Form I-9 lists on the back documents that are acceptable proof of identity and right to work. An immigrant worker must have a work permit and a Social Security number.

- Verify all new hires, not just those you think may be foreign, by completing the I-9 form.
- Complete the I-9 form after the person is hired, within three days of hire.
- Don't ask to see work papers at the time of the job interview.
- Tell applicants you must check new employees' work papers after they are hired.
- Let the worker decide which identity and work papers to show you. It's illegal to ask for more or different documents.
- Accept any document listed on the back of the I-9 that appears genuine. You don't have to be a document expert.

You can obtain the *Handbook for Employers,* which includes copies of Form I-9 and instructions for filling it out, by writing the U.S. Department of Justice, Immigration and Naturalization Service, 425 I Street, NW, Washington, DC 20536. If you have questions, call the 24-hour Employment Eligibility Hotline at 1-800-777-7700. Or, the form and handbook can be obtained from your local INS office.

For a free copy of the brochure, *Employer's Guide to Hiring Immigrants and Other Workers,* call or write Office of the Special Counsel, U.S. Department of Justice, P.O. Box 65490, Washington, DC 20035-5490, 1-800-255-7688. This document discusses the I-9 process and provides specific details on the most common legal documents that employees may show to prove they may work legally in the U.S.

Would-be employers of home caregivers must recognize that their responsibilities go beyond honoring, respecting and caring about their employees. The hard fact is that they must comply with the labor and tax laws established by state and federal agencies to regulate in-home employment.

The goal of this book is to encourage and support you in taking on this responsibility yourself. To be most prudent, you may find it reassuring to let your accountant and/or insurance agent review your efforts, at least for the first go-around. When you are confident that your arrangement is sound, you are free to concentrate on the primary goal of consumer-directed home care: the best quality of life for the elder(s) in your family.

EMPLOYEE FILE CARD

Employee's Name_____

Home Address_____

Telephone_____

Social Security Number_____ Date of Birth _____

Start Date_____ End Date_____

Reason for leaving

NOTE: For more detailed help in locating tax information and publications, please see Appendix A. Details on the IRS "Tele-Tax" information system are given in Appendix B.

Chapter Eleven

AGENCY-DIRECTED HOME CARE

"My caregiving experience was over thirteen years — including a mother with cancer and Alzheimer's and a stroke victim husband. I had them both at the same time, twenty-four hours a day.

How I wished for a respite, a friend I could talk to without thinking I was bellyaching, a chance to walk away and just kick rocks in the river. A hand to hold, a shoulder to lean on ..."

— Freda Garner, Secretary, age 62

HOME CARE AGENCIES COME IN A VAST ASSORTMENT OF shapes and sizes. These agencies can serve as the source of nurses, social workers, rehabilitative therapists, dieticians and/or home caregivers. They can provide home services ranging from housecleaning to bed baths. The list of possible services is almost limitless.

Home care agencies are operated by private, nonprofit groups (Visiting Nurses Association, health and social service agencies), proprietary/commercial concerns (Kelly Assisted Living, Interim), or governmental entities (public health department). The following simplified chart categorizes the basic types of agencies:

TYPES OF HOME CARE AGENCIES

Medicare-certified home health agency

Medicare pays?	Yes
Skilled care?	Yes
Semi-skilled care?	Yes

Private-pay home health agency

Medicare pays?	No
Skilled care?	Yes
Semi-skilled care?	Yes

Homemaker/home care agency

Medicare pays?	No
Skilled care?	No
Semi-skilled care?	Yes

Should I Use a Home Care Agency?

Why use an agency rather than contracting privately? For one thing, agencies can provide a comprehensive menu of services under one roof, from personal care to skilled nursing to specialized rehabilitative therapies. Easy access to an array of services, ranging from the simplest to the most medically-oriented and technically advanced, can be a tremendous advantage in some cases.

A team of agency workers can help families maintain a difficult-to-care-for elder at home without encountering "burnout," a very common symptom of caregiving caused by excessive demands. Burnout negatively impacts motivation, behavior, attitude and the quality of caregiving. To be most effective and to avoid burnout, a home care worker must also have respite, reprieve and assistance. This is exactly what a team of agency workers can provide.

Agency workers can also be a godsend when your home caregiver doesn't show up for work due to illness, car trouble or family emergencies. An agency is often able to dispatch a replacement immediately. Having such an agency safety net offers the flexibility you need to make a consumer-directed care plan work over the long term. In other words, you may find that you end up using neither agency-directed nor consumer-directed home care exclusively, but instead use a "mixed mode" approach.

There is no question that purchasing services from an agency saves paperwork and time, and can provide reliable and trustworthy help. The benefits of letting someone else handle the taxes, record keeping, background screening, and all the other responsibilities of the employer role may be especially appealing if you need to hire two or more workers. The cost, convenience, legal responsibilities and overall risk factors must be balanced for your best interest.

Getting Agency Services Started

You will usually be asked to sign one or more forms in order to get home care started. These may include: a consent agreement, release of medical information forms, a service contract or letter outlining services to be provided, costs and payment obligations and financial or insurance disclosure authorizations.

The agency maintains all responsibility for personnel records, payroll, insurance and Social Security taxes. Time slips are provided for your review.

If your elder qualifies for home care according to Medicare guidelines, the agency will bill the government directly. You'll pay nothing for Medicare-covered services, and just 20% of the approved amount for covered medical equipment. Otherwise (non-Medicare), the agency will bill you and/or your insurance company on a regular basis.

How Can I Select the Best Agency?

It's important to shop for a home care agency as carefully as you would for a doctor or lawyer. This is a daunting proposition however, because the industry has no universally accepted standards of care. Agencies can, however, earn a "seal of approval" by adopting the standards set by the accreditation bodies listed in Appendix G. Accreditation is one indicator of service quality.

After you've determined if an agency possesses any required state license(s), accreditation from a recognized national organization, and/or any additional documents, your best approach is to verify the agency's *local reputation*. In an industry in which standards can vary widely, reputation may be the best yardstick of quality.

Start by asking your doctor for his recommendation. Hospital discharge planners, social workers or geriatric care managers can also point you in the right direction. These pros generally have a good handle on who's doing a good job and who's not. And, don't forget to ask for recommendations from your friends who have used a home care agency in the past.

Once you narrow your choices, contact your local Better Business Bureau or consumer protection office to learn more about the agencies that interest you. One expert suggests that if an agency has been in business for ten years or more, and has no serious complaints on file, it can be considered a strong candidate.

In addition, you can check with your state or regional Long Term Care Ombudsman Program, a little-known but useful consumer watchdog service. Until recently, local ombudsman programs mainly dealt with consumerism in relation to nursing homes, with citizen activists — termed "ombudsmen" — investigating complaints made by or on behalf of patients. Ombudsman programs are now beginning to extend their range into the arena of home care. If you would like to learn more about ombudsman services in relation to home care agencies, use the Eldercare Locator to contact the program nearest you. (See Appendix B for more information on the Eldercare Locator.)

Does Medicare Pay For Home Care?

A Medicare beneficiary — either because of age or disability — may be entitled to home health care benefits at no personal cost. The key to receiving coverage (skilled nursing, skilled therapy services, home health aide services) is being physically homebound and requiring a *skilled medical service*. For those who meet these criteria, a physician will normally write out the order that qualifies the patient for Medicare-reimbursable home health care. The physician's order opens the door to Medicare reimbursement for skilled nursing care at home, and, in addition makes paraprofessional and social work services available during the period that skilled nursing care is rendered.

If your elder's care is to be paid by Medicare, make sure the agency you deal with is *Medicare-certified.* (Medicare certification simply means that the agency has voluntarily met certain minimum standards in order to participate in this government program.) Unless you check first, you may find yourself needlessly paying bills out-of-pocket.

Other public and private programs that can help cover costs of home care include Medicaid, private health insurance and health maintenance organizations (HMOs). Additionally, the Veterans Administration will pay for home health assistance when the condition is connected to military service (refer to Chapter Three).

Your family's out-of-pocket cost for home care will depend on the elder's medical status and whether any health insurances are applicable to the specific health condition.

It is important to understand that Medicare *never* pays for health care workers to "stay" with a patient over the long term. Care is on a *temporary basis* for *rehabilitative* care. Under Medicare, frequency of services will decrease as the patient improves. If the patient does not improve, Medicare-reimbursed home health care allows time for other arrangements to be made; it is *not* long-term care.

Many of the services provided by a Medicare-certified home care agency are available to consumers without a doctor's order; however, without an order from the doctor, services are generally not reimbursable by Medicare or other third-party payors. In other words, payment will be out-of-pocket, from the family's income or assets. Of course, if you wish to arrange home care directly (without a doctor's order), you are not limited to Medicare-certified agencies. Simply call any home care agency (Medicare-certified, private pay or homemaker/home care) and request the service you need.

The Home Care Team

The home care "team" includes a variety of caregivers, from in-home employees all the way to physicians. Here's a brief roster:

Physicians (MDs and DOs) may prescribe home care. They have the authority to choose which types of workers will be assigned, and for how long.

Registered Nurses (RNs) do everything from changing dressings and giving injections to noting the patient's condition in reports to the doctor.

Licensed Practical Nurses (LPNs) work under the supervision of an RN or physician; duties differ from state to state.

Social Workers provide counseling, find and coordinate resources and sometimes supervise home care services.

Registered Dieticians (RDs) plan and monitor special diets related to health.

Speech Therapists assist with communications problems, such as learning to speak after a stroke.

Respiratory Therapists help patients cope with breathing difficulties.

Physical Therapists help patients in regaining lost physical abilities or gaining new skills.

Home Health Aides are paraprofessionals who assist with personal care activities, and may do housework; they may administer oral medications under the supervision of an R.N.

Homemakers assist with cleaning, laundry and shopping; their responsibilities are restricted to housework.

How To Evaluate Home Care Agencies
No elder or family should feel obligated to put up with unsatisfactory home care. Competition for dollars in the home care industry is fierce, and most agencies will go out of their way to keep their customers happy.

Selecting an agency can be likened to choosing any other kind of personal/professional service. You need to look below the surface by carefully checking reputation, credentials, experience and range of services offered.

Try to plan ahead. Make phone calls, make visits, and ask the hard questions. Get a clear picture of all the costs and make sure that there are no extra, hidden or add-on fees.

Use the following checklist to evaluate an agency's performance. The checklist was developed by Liz Williams, Community Senior Care Coordinator, The Palms at Largo, Largo, Florida.

EVALUATING HOME CARE AGENCIES: A CHECKLIST

☐ When you call the office, are phones answered with a friendly voice within three rings?

☐ When asking about costs and services, do you receive the information needed to satisfy your individual questions?

☐ Do staff arrive promptly at the time of their scheduled appointment?

☐ Do staff identify themselves at the door?

☐ Are staff competent and skillful with the elder's care?

☐ Do staff explain the care they are going to give before performing the services?

☐ Does the bill for services accurately state the cost of services provided?

☐ Are questions about your bill answered satisfactorily with adequate and accurate information?

Remember that you are making a choice that will directly and personally impact the quality of an elder's life!

Commercial Chains

Large home health agency chains are listed below. You are likely to find a branch office of one of these national corporations in your community. Call them to find the phone numbers of the offices most convenient to you, or check the Yellow Pages under "Home Health Services" for other local or regional agencies.

First American Home Care *(the largest privately owned, Medicare-certified home health provider in the U.S.)*
3528 Darien Highway
P.O. Box 1056
Brunswick, GA 31521
(800) 777-6876

Interim Health Care *(affiliated with H&R Block)*
8616 Griffin Road, Cooper City, FL 33328
(305) 434-0300

Staff Builders Home Health Care *(established by the Staff Builders temporary-worker agency)*
1981 Marcus Avenue, Lake Success, NY 11042
(516) 358-1000

Kelly Assisted Living Services *(Kelly Services, Inc. subsidiary)*
999 West Big Beaver Road, Troy, MI 48084
(800) 541-9818, (313) 362-4444

EPILOGUE

IN THE COURSE OF WRITING THIS BOOK, I HAD OCCASION TO TEST its usefulness in my own family. My 87-year-old Uncle Jackson of San Antonio, Texas had a stroke nine months ago. His saga since has been a success story and he has consented to allow me to share it.

My deceased father's eldest brother is slim and erect and looks as if a map of Texas is imprinted upon his weathered face. He has adjusted quite well since the death of his wife about seven years ago. He moved from his family home into a condominium in San Antonio to be closer to his woman friend, the absolutely beautiful 80-year-old widow of an army general. Up until his stroke, Uncle Jackson lived very well: he drove a pick-up truck, went to church every Sunday, rode his bicycle around the neighborhood and squired "Mrs. Van Wagner" to local social functions.

The stroke happened as strokes typically do, suddenly and terrifyingly, striking in the middle of the night. Uncle Jackson had wisely purchased an emergency alert response system so was able to press a button for help as he lay immobilized on the floor. Paramedics were there in a matter of minutes to transport him to a major hospital, where he received acute medical care for about three-and-a-half weeks.

Uncle Jackson has outlived most of his brothers and sisters and other family members. His one surviving sibling, my Aunt Opal, aged 76, traveled immediately to be with him in the hospital. Although she couldn't stay with him for the entire time, she made visits every weekend to manage his household and to begin to coordinate with the rest of the family to plan for his long-term care. She was quite concerned that my Uncle might never be able to return home.

Although the stroke was termed "light," I would hate to have seen a heavy one. Uncle Jackson could barely talk, nor could he move the right side of his upper body. And, most distressingly, he seemed to be suffering a great deal of emotional upset; he often became distraught and tearful as I tried to communicate with him over the phone in the early days of his hospitalization.

In time, however, Uncle Jackson was discharged to a rehab center for a short period of speech and physical therapy. As he struggled to recover from the effects of his stroke, his progress was slow and painful but very real, with steady improvements that were met with surprise and delight by all who know him. He was quite adamant at the rehab center that his main goal in life was to return to his small apartment to continue living as he always had — independently. That is when I decided I had better fly out to Texas and start trying to help him set up in-home help.

I stayed at Uncle Jackson's house for about four days while he was still at the rehab center. I had remained in close contact with him and my aunt throughout the hospitalization, but some things have to be done on the scene. As as professional gerontologist I have a good familiarity with aging services and felt my best bet was to start by making a visit to the local senior center. This proved to be a good idea as I was able to identify the full range of local social services in a "one-stop shopping" kind of visit. The center director actually remembered my

Uncle, having recently enlisted him as a recipient of Meals-on-Wheels. She was saddened to hear about his stroke and took it on as a personal mission to help me help him during my short visit.

Probably the most valuable thing I obtained at the senior center was a three-page typed listing of women in the local area who were looking for jobs as in-home caregivers. I went back to the apartment and immediately began to start calling names on the list. My job was made a lot easier by the director, who had alerted me to the three or four women she thought would be most appropriate for work with my Uncle.

Uncle Jackson was able to come home for three or four hours a day during my stay, and we interviewed potential home caregivers together. The only likely applicant we met with, however, brought her little puppy to the interview and it was very clear that she and the dog were inseparable; obviously it would accompany her on any of her in-home assignments. Although my Uncle is an extremely loving man, he's not the worlds' greatest pet lover, so that immediately disqualified this otherwise very promising candidate.

I began to feel that our efforts would be unsuccessful and that perhaps I would have to recruit a worker through an agency, at least for the short term. Although I considered that less desirable, from both relationship and financial standpoints, it did offer peace of mind as a short-term solution.

When the time came for me to return to work, no caregiver had been found and Uncle Jackson was still in the rehab center. With help from my Aunt, however, he was able to continue the recruiting process. They found and hired a "gem of a lady" (his words): a married woman of 51 who has lived in the local community since her childhood. She has a high school education and knows a great many of my Uncle's fellow San Antonians.

"Mrs. Basta" comes six hours a day from 8:30 to 2:30, five days a week. My Uncle pays her $6.00 per hour (other workers in his area with similar jobs are paid as high as $8.00 an hour). Although she is a smoker, my Uncle won't let her smoke in the house; he is quite concerned as to what she will do when the weather turns cold. She is good at housekeeping but is an even better cook. Since she started my Uncle has gained about ten pounds, mostly by feasting on daily noon meals of steaks, pork chops and center-cut ham slices. (His doctor is tolerant, though not pleased!)

I asked Uncle Jackson what he likes about Mrs. Basta. Other than raving about her good cooking, he mentioned that she does things around his house the way she might do them at home. I asked for an example and he said, "Well, she went into my bathroom and cleaned all by brushes and combs, soaking them in soapy water and scrubbing them together until they were like new." And without being asked.

Another wonderful service Mrs. Basta provides is transporting my Uncle in her own car. She takes him to his bank, to his barber shop, and to the grocery store. Although he often waits in the car, the outings make a nice change of scenery for him. He likes to prepare the grocery list with her and then go over her purchases as she loads them into the car. They have worked out a good system toether; she uses about $30 worth of cash; he checks her purchases against the receipt, and she returns the change.

My uncle is a very meticulous person, and he has painstakingly maintained wage and hour records so he can pay the correct amount of Social Security taxes. He did share with me what a "lot of damn trouble" this record-keeping is and how glad he will be when it no longer has to be done every three months but just once a year.

Uncle Jackson continues to make a remarkable recovery from his stroke. In many ways of course, he will never be the

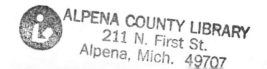

same. He has had to give up driving, and has sold his beloved truck. His energy level is extremely low and his letters are now written in a crabbed-looking hand. On the plus side, his speech has improved remarkably and he is still seeing Mrs. Van Wagner regularly and sending me glowing reports about Mrs. Basta and their wonderful meals together.

Since my uncle is an old fashioned gentleman, uncomfortable discussing personal matters, I was unable to gather much information about the kinds of personal care that his home caregiver provides. Given the nature of his stroke and his impaired mobility, I believe that the care must be somewhat extensive, involving the laying out of clothes, help in prepration for personal grooming and similar activities. Whatever the true extent of help, I'm comfortable knowing that the housework is being done, groceries are being bought, errands are run, and my Uncle is well and happy.

In many ways this arrangement feels precarious. We still have no backup for Mrs. Basta for her vacation times or in the event of her illness. But, it is working, and my dear, distinguished, proud Uncle continues to be the patriarch of his neighborhood and the king of his home.

I wish a similar success story to the elder(s) in your family

— D. Helen Susik
1995

Appendices

TAX INFORMATION AND PUBLICATIONS

Each year the IRS prepares updated publications which can answer many of your tax questions and help you prepare your annual federal tax return. All of these publications are free and readily obtainable. The following sources provide both publications and federal tax forms.

Local public libraries. Your library generally maintains reference copies throughout the year of the most frequently requested publications and forms. You can photocopy any of the available forms or publications if the library does not have additional copies to give out.

Local IRS offices. These offices can answer your tax questions. They also maintain almost every publication and form that the IRS publishes. If you live in an area where a local IRS office is not available to answer your tax questions, call **1-800-829-1040.**

IRS Forms and Publications Telephone Center. The IRS maintains a nationwide toll-free telephone ordering center throughout the year. You can call **1-800-829-3676** to obtain any form or publication currently available. Your material will arrive approximately seven to ten working days after you place your order. Use this toll-free number only to request information on forms and publications; if you have tax questions, call 800-829-1040.

IRS mail-order distribution centers. You can order through the mail any form or publication published by the IRS.

If you live in:
Alaska, Arizona, California, Colorado, Hawaii, Idaho, Kansas, Montana, New Mexico, Nevada, Oklahoma, Oregon, Utah, Washington, Wyoming
Write to:
Western Area Distribution Center
IRS Forms
Rancho Cordova, CA 95743-0001

If you live in:
Alabama, Arkansas, Illinois, Indiana, Iowa, Kentucky, Louisiana, Michigan, Minnesota, Mississippi, Missouri, Nebraska, North Dakota, Ohio, South Dakota, Tennessee, Texas, Wisconsin
Write to:
Central Area Distribution Center
IRS Forms
P.O. Box 8903
Bloomington, IL 61702-8903

If you live in:
Connecticut, Delaware, District of Columbia, Florida, Georgia, Maine, Maryland, Massachusetts, New Hampshire, New Jersey, New York, North Carolina, Pennsylvania, Rhode Island, South Carolina, Vermont, Virginia, West Virginia
Write to:
Eastern Area Distribution Center
IRS Forms
P.O. Box 25866
Richmond, VA 23261-5074

Individuals who are deaf or hearing impaired and have access to TDD equipment should call the following toll-free number for assistance: **1-800-829-4059**

THE IRS "TELE-TAX" INFORMATION SYSTEM

The IRS now provides recorded tax information to answer many Federal tax questions. You can listen to up to three topics on each call you make.

A list of topics related to hiring home helpers is listed below. Touch-tone service is available 24 hours a day, seven days a week.

Select, by number, the topic you want to hear. Then, call the appropriate phone number listed on the next pages. Have paper and pen handy to take notes.

Topic No.	Subject
	Employer Tax Information
751	Social Security and Medicare withholding rates
752	Form W-2 — Where, when, and how to file
753	Form W-4 — Employee's Withholding Allowance Certificate
755	Employer identification number (EIN) — How to apply
756	Employment taxes for household employees
757	Form 941 — Deposit requirements
758	Form 941 — Employer's Quarterly Federal Tax Return
759	Form 940/940-EZ — Deposit requirements
760	Form 940/940-EZ — Employer's Annual Federal Unemployment Tax Return

Topic numbers are effective January 1, 1994

Appendix C

ELDERCARE LOCATOR

The Administration on Aging (AoA), the National Association of Area Agencies on Aging (NAAAA), and the National Association of State Units on Aging (NASUA) are working together on a National Information and Referral (I&R) Initiative to help link older persons and their families to information and resources.

Through the National I&R Initiative's toll-free **Eldercare Locator,** individuals have access to more than 4,800 state and local information and referral service providers, identified for every ZIP code in the country. The database also includes special purpose I&R telephone numbers for:

- Alzheimer's hotlines
- Adult day care/respite services
- Nursing home/ombudsman assistance
- Consumer fraud
- Hospital/nursing home information
- In-home care complaints
- Legal services
- Elder abuse/protective services
- Medicaid/Medigap information
- Tax assistance
- Transportation

The **Eldercare Locator, 1-800-677-1116,** is available weekdays, 9:00 a.m. to 11:00 p.m. (EST).

Additional information about the National I&R Initiative or the **Eldercare Locator** can be obtained by contacting the National Association of Area Agencies on Aging.

AREA AGENCIES ON AGING

Created in 1973 under the Older Americans Act, the Area Agencies on Aging address the specific needs and concerns of all Americans over 60. As the third member of the government's "aging network" which also includes the federal Administration on Aging (AoA) and the state units or commissions on aging (offices also exist for D.C. and the U.S. territories) each of the over 670 Area Agencies on Aging (also known as County Offices on Aging) throughout the U.S. is responsible for a single city, county, or multi-county district.

Funded by the Older Americans Act, state and local governments and private contributions, each Area Agency on Aging provides services, directly and indirectly, that are tailored to the needs of its particular community.

Most services provided through your local Area Agency on Aging are free; others have a very minimal charge. While the specific services they provide vary from area to area, all Agencies on Aging provide:

In-Home Services. These may include:
- Home-delivered meals (known as meals-on-wheels) which help older people maintain an adequate diet
- Homemaker and chore services, including light house-keeping, laundry, shopping, errands, and meal preparation
- In-home health and personal care
- Daily visits or phone calls to elderly persons who live alone
- Support services, like counseling and rehabilitation
- Respite care to relieve caregivers for short periods each day
- Home maintenance, repairs, and weatherization for those who are unable or cannot afford to take care of their homes

Community Services. These may include:
- Multi-purpose senior centers
- Adult day care
- Communal meals
- Adult protective services for older persons abused by others in their household
- Legal aid and tax assistance
- Counseling on available community services
- Recreation and rehabilitation
- Employment services, including job training and job search assistance

Access Services. In addition to its role as a clearinghouse for information and referrals in a community, the Agency may provide services like:
- Transportation of older people to nutrition and meal sites, medical appointments, and shopping areas
- Individual case management
- Assistance finding housing alternatives in the community, such as housemate matching services
- Outreach programs for needy seniors who may be eligible for Supplemental Security Income, Medicaid, food stamps, and other programs designed to aid individuals
-

Services for Individuals in Long-Term Care Facilities. These may include:
- Individual counseling in the facility
- Case work
- Visitation
- Escorts to activities outside the facility
- Transportation of handicapped seniors to services outside the facility
- Ombudsman services to help ensure proper care of individuals in the facility, and to help resolve complaints about the facility or care received

Appendix E

THE AGING NETWORK

The Older Americans Act was enacted in 1965 to develop a federal-state-community framework for a service system responsive to the needs of older persons. Called the "aging network," this system now includes:

- **The Administration on Aging (AoA).** A federal agency that provides information about social services, nutrition, education, senior centers and other services for older Americans.

  Administration on Aging, Office on External Affairs
  330 Independence Avenue, S.W.
  Washington, DC 20201
  (202) 619-0724

- **State Units on Aging. SUAs** are designated by law as the state-level focal point for all activities related to the needs of and services for older Americans.

  The National Association of State Units on Aging
  1225 I Street, N.W., Suite 725
  Washington, DC 20005
  (202) 898-2578

Area Agencies on Aging. AAAs now number more than 670 and cover all parts of the United States. A large part of their budgets comes from the Older Americans Act, but the AAAs are likely to tap other public, and some private, sources of funds. AAAs serve as the local entities that plan services for seniors and administer provisions of the Older Americans Act within their communities.

> The National Association of Area Agencies on Aging
> 1112 16th Street, N.W., Suite 100
> Washington, D.C. 20006
> (202) 296-8130

- **Community-based Service Providers.** State and area agencies are in close contact with service providers, who put Older Americans Act funds to widely varying uses.

STATE UNITS ON AGING

ALABAMA
Commission on Aging,
770 Washington Avenue, Suite 470, RSA Plaza
Montgomery, AL 36130
Phone: 205-242-5743

ALASKA
Older Alaskans Commission
Department of Administration
Pouch C, Mail Station 0209
Juneau, AK 99811-0209
Phone: 907-465-3250

ARIZONA
Aging and Adult Administration
Deparment of Economic Security
1789 W. Jefferson St., #950A
Phoenix, AZ 85007
Phone: 602-542-4446

ARKANSAS
Division of Aging and Adult Services
Department of Human Services
7th and Main Street
Little Rock, AR 72203
Phone: 501-682-2441

CALIFORNIA
Department of Aging
1600 K Street
Sacramento, CA 95814
Phone: 916-322-5290

COLORADO
Aging and Adult Services
Department of Social Services
1575 Sherman Street, 4th Floor
Denver, CO 80203
Phone: 303-866-3851

CONNECTICUT
Connecticut Department on Aging
175 Main Street
Hartford, CT 06106
Phone: 203-566-3238

DELAWARE
Division of Aging, Department of Health & Social Services
1901 N. DuPont Highway
New Castle, DE 19720
Phone: 302-577-4791

DISTRICT OF COLUMBIA
D.C. Office on Aging
One Judiciary Square
441 4th Street N.W, 9th Floor
Washington, DC 20001
Phone: 202-724-5622

FLORIDA
Department of Elder Affairs,
1317 Winewood Blvd., Bldg. 1, Room 317
Tallahassee, FL 32399
Phone: 904-922-5297

GEORGIA
Office on Aging
#2 Peachtree Street NE, 18th Floor
Atlanta, GA 30303
Phone: 404-657-5258

HAWAII
Executive Office on Aging, Office of the Governor
335 Merchant Street, Suite 241
Honolulu, HI 96813
Phone: 808-586-0100

IDAHO
Office on Aging
Room 108, Statehouse
Boise, ID 83720
Phone: 208-334-3833

ILLINOIS
Illinois Department on Aging
421 East Capital Avenue
Springfield, IL 62701
Phone: 217-785-2870

INDIANA
Bureau of Aging/In-Home Services
402 W. Washington Street, E-431
Indianapolis, IN 46207
Phone: 317-232-7020

IOWA
Iowa Department of Elder Affairs
914 Grand Avenue, Suite 236 - Jewett Bldg.
Des Moines, IA 50319
Phone: 515-281-5187

KANSAS
Department on Aging
Docking State Office Building, 122-S
915 SW Harrison St.
Topeka, KS 66612
Phone: 913-296-4986

KENTUCKY
Division of Aging Services, Cabinet for Human Resources
275 East Main Street
6 West, Frankfort, KY 40621
Phone: 502-564-6930

LOUISIANA
Office of Elderly Affairs
4550 North Boulevard, 2nd Floor
Baton Rouge, LA 70806
Phone: 504-925-1700

MAINE
Bureau of Elder and Adult Services
Department of Human Services
State House, Station #11
Augusta, ME 04333
Phone: 207-626-5335

MARYLAND
Maryland Office on Aging
State Office Building
301 W. Preston Street, Room 1004
Baltimore, MD 21201
Phone: 401-225-1100

MASSACHUSETTS
Executive Office of Elder Affairs
1 Ashburton Place, 5th Floor
Boston, MA 02108
Phone: 617-727-7750

MICHIGAN
Office of Services to the Aging
PO Box 30026
Lansing, MI 48909
Phone: 517-373-8230

MINNESOTA
Board on Aging
444 Lafayette Road
St. Paul, MN 55155
Phone: 612-296-2770

MISSISSIPPI
Council on Aging, Divison of Aging & Adult Services
750 N. State Street
Jackson, MS 39203
Phone: 601-359-4929

MISSOURI
Division on Aging, Department of Social Services
615 Howerton Court
Jefferson City, MO 65102
Phone: 314-751-3082

MONTANA
The Governor's Office on Aging
State Capitol Building, Capitol Station, Room 219
Helena, MT 59620
Phone: 406-444-3111

NEBRASKA
Nebraska Department on Aging
301 Centennial Mall, South
Lincoln, NE 68509
Phone: 402-471-2306

NEVADA
Division for Aging Services
445 Apple Street, Suite 114
Las Vegas, NV 89502
Phone: 702-688-2964

NEW HAMPSHIRE
Division of Elderly & Adult Services
State Office Park South, 115 Pleasant Street, Annex Bldg. #1
Concord, NH 03301
Phone: 603-271-4680

NEW JERSEY
Division on Aging, Department of Community Affairs
CN807, South Broad and Front Streets
Trenton, NJ 08625
Phone: 609-292-4833

NEW MEXICO
State Agency on Aging
La Villa Rivera Bldg., 224 E. Palace Avenue
Santa Fe, NM 87501
Phone: 505-827-7640

NEW YORK
New York State Office for the Aging
New York State Plaza, Agency Bldg. #2
Albany, NY 12223
Phone: 518-474-4425

NORTH CAROLINA
Division on Aging
693 Palmer Drive
Raleigh, NC 27626
Phone: 919-733-3983

NORTH DAKOTA
Aging Services Division, Department of Human Services
1929 N. Washington Street
Bismark, ND 58507-7070
Phone: 701-224-2577

OHIO
Ohio Department of Aging
50 W. Broad Street, 9th Floor
Columbus, OH 43266
Phone: 614-466-5500

OKLAHOMA
Aging Services Division, Department of Human Services
312 North East 28th St.
Oklahoma City, OK 73125
Phone: 405-521-2327

OREGON
Senior & Disabled Services Division
500 Summer Street NE, 2nd Floor N.
Salem, OR 97310
Phone: 503-378-4728

PENNSYLVANIA
Department of Aging
Market Street State Office Bldg. 400 Market Street, 7th Floor
Harrisburg, PA 17101
Phone: 717-783-1550

RHODE ISLAND
Department of Elderly Affairs
160 Pine Street
Providence, RI 02903
Phone: 401-277-2858

SOUTH CAROLINA
Division on Aging
202 Arbor Lake Dr., #301
Columbia, SC 29223
Phone: 803-735-7500

SOUTH DAKOTA
Office of Adult Services and Aging
Kneip Bldg., 700 Governors Drive
Pierre, SD 57501
Phone: 605-773-3656

TENNESSEE
Tennessee Commission on Aging
706 Church Street, Suite 201
Nashville, TN 37243
Phone: 615-741-2056

TEXAS
Department on Aging
1949 IH-35 South
Austin, TX 78741
Phone: 512-444-2727

UTAH
Division of Aging and Adult Services, Dept. of Human Services
120 North 200 West
Salt Lake City, UT 84145-0500
Phone: 801-538-3910

VERMONT
Department of Aging and Disabilities
103 S. Main Street
Waterbury, VT 05671-2301
Phone: 802-241-2400

VIRGINIA
Virginia Department for the Aging
700 East Franklin Street, 10th Floor
Richmond, VA 23219
Phone: 804-225-2271

WASHINGTON
Aging & Adult Services Administration
Department of Social & Health Services
PO Box 45600
Olympia, WA 98504-5600
Phone: 206-586-3768

WEST VIRGINIA
Commission on Aging
Holly Grove, 1900 Kamawha Blvd.
East Charleston, WV 25305
Phone: 304-558-3317

WISCONSIN
Bureau on Aging, Division of Community Services
217 S. Hamilton Street, Suite 300
Madison, WI 53707
Phone: 608-266-2536

WYOMING
Wyoming Division on Aging
Wyoming Department of Health
Hathaway Bldg., Room 139
Cheyenne, WY 82002
Phone: 307-777-7986

CHAPTER RESOURCES

Chapter One — You're the Boss!

Alliance for Aging Research
21 K Street, NW, Suite 305
Washington, DC 20006
(202)-293-2856
The Alliance is a leading citizen advocacy organization for promoting scientific research to ensure healthy aging.

Eldercare America, Inc.
1141 Loxford Terrace
Silver Spring, MD 20901
(301) 593-1621
Represents the interests of caregivers by promoting favorable legislation and programs. Produces videos about caregiving that may be purchased.

National Family Caregivers Association
9621 East Bexhill Drive
Kensington, MD 20895-3104
(301) 942-6430
The NFCA strives to meet the needs of family caregivers and to improve the caregiveer's quality of life through a quarterly newsletter, a person-to-person network and educational materials for caregivers.

Older Women's League
666 11th Street NW, Suite 700
Washington, DC 20001
(202) 783-6686
A National membership organization formed to provide mutual support for midlife and older women and caregivers. Write for a listing of publications.

Chapter 2 — The Role and Cost of Home Caregivers

American Association of Retired Persons (AARP)
601 E Street NW
Washington, DC 20049
(202) 434-2277

AARP Publications:
To order any free single copy of these AARP resources, send a request listing the title and stock number to AARP Fulfillment Section. Allow 6 to 8 weeks for delivery.

A Handbook About Care In the Home (Stock #D955). 24-page handbook. Discusses arranging for and evaluating home care services; reviews the types of home care services.

Care Management: Arranging for Long Term Care (Stock #D15803). Describes how care management can be used to locate and arrange long term care services.

Making Wise Decisions for Long Term Care (Stock #D12435). A guide to long term care services and financing.

Staying At Home: A Guide to Long-Term Care and Housing (Stock #D14986)

Your Home, Your Choice (Stock #D12143).

Children of Aging Parents
Woodbourne Office Campus, Suite 302-A, Dept. MC
1609 Woodbourne Road
Levittown, PA 19057
(215) 945-6900
Children of Aging Parents (CAPS) provides information and referrals to national caregiver resources; has developed and maintains caregiver support groups, and publishes a national newsletter containing up-to-date information for caregivers. Ask for their "Medicare/Medicaid Fact Sheet." Include a stamped self-addressed legal envelope when writing. You may also wish to order the Care Sharing Directory, *a national directory of private geriatric care managers.*

United Seniors Health Cooperative
1331 H Street, NW, Suite 500
Washington, DC 20005
(202) 393-6222
This cooperative publishes a variety of books of interest to consumers of homecare, including Long-term Care: A Dollar and Sense Guide.

Chapter 3 — A Home Caregiver for Me?

Aging Network Services
4400 East-West Highway, Suite 907
Bethesda, MD 20814
(301) 657-4329
A national network of over 300 geriatric social workers in private practice. This agency requires members to have professional credentials and licenses, plus care management experience.

Association of Jewish Family and Children's Agencies
Elder Support Network
(800) 634-7346
The network has a link between families and older relatives through Jewish Family Service Agencies.

National Association of Area Agencies on Aging
1112 - 16th Street NW, Suite 100
Washington, DC 20036
(202) 296-8130
Publishes a list of AAAs who offer care management services.

National Association of Professional Geriatric Care Managers
1604 N. Country Club Road
Tucson, AZ 85716
(602) 881-8008
Publishes a directory of professional geriatric care managers ($35.00). Makes referrals to private geriatric care managers with college degrees and at least two years of geriatric experience.

National Association of Social Workers
7 50 First Street NE, Suite 700
Washington, DC 20002
(800) 638-8799
Publishes professional standards for social work care management.

Chapter 4 — Recruiting Your Helper

National Displaced Homemaker Network
1625 K Street, NW, Suite 300
Washington, DC 20006
(202) 467-6346
Nationwide referral for displaced homemakers seeking employment and training services.

National Health Information Center (NHIC)
PO Box 1133
Washington, DC 20013-1133
(800) 336-4797
NHIC is a free service of the Office of Disease Prevention and Health Promotion, U.S. Public Health Service. It is a central source of information and referral for any kind of health question, including identification of national and local health organizations and programs. NHIC maintains a library and a computer database of over 2,000 health-related organizations.

National Hospice Organization
1901 N-Moore Street, Suite 901
Arlington, VA 22209
800-658-8898
The NHO publishes various informational pamphlets as well as an annual Guide to The Nation's Hospices

National Interfaith Coalition on Aging
c/o National Council on Aging
409 Third Street, SW
Washington, DC 20024
(202) 479-1200
NICA is a nondenominational, nonprofit organization created as a resource for religious workers and groups who work with older Americans. Local chapters may represent a source of volunteer in-home assistance.

Chapter 5 — Selecting Your Caregiver

National Eldercare Institute on Long Term Care and Alzheimer's Disease
University of South Florida
Suncoast Gerontology Center MDC Box 50
Tampa, FL 33612-4799
(813) 974-4355
The Institute publishes articles and a service of free consumer-oriented "Agelines" on issues related to aging and long term care.

General Organizational Resources:

Alzheimer's Disease & Related Disorders Association
919 N. Michigan Avenue, Suite 1000, Chicago, IL 60611-1676
(800) 272-3900

American Cancer Society
77 E. Monroe, 13th Floor, Chicago, IL 60603
(800) 227-2345

Arthritis Foundation
1314 Spring Street, Atlanta, GA 30309
(800) 283-7800

American Diabetes Association
1660 Duke Street, Alexandria, VA 22314
(800) 232-3472

American Foundation for the Blind
15 West 16th Street
New York, NY 10011
(800) AFB-LIND

American Heart Association
9933 Lawler, Room 430, Skokie, IL 60077
(708) 675-1535

American Lung Association
1740 Broadway, New York, NY 10019
(212) 315-8700

Arthritis Foundation
1314 Spring Street, NW, Atlanta, GA 30309
(800) 283-7800

Chapter 6 — Running Background Checks

AARP Criminal Justice Services, Code GS
1901 K Street NW, Washington, DC 20049
(202) 872-4700

National Council Against Health Fraud
PO Box 33008, Kansas City, MO 64114

National Council on Independent Living
310 S. Peoria Street, Ste. 201, Chicago, IL 60607
(312) 226-1006

National Crime Prevention Council
733 15th Street NW, Ste. 540, Washington, DC 20005
(202) 393-7141

National Organization for Victim Assistance
717 D Street NW, Washington, DC 20531
(202) 393-6682

National Safety Council
1121 Spring Lake Drive, Itasca, IL 60143
(708) 285-1121

Chapter 7 — Completing the Employment Agreement

Brookdale Center on Aging
Institute on Law and Rights of Older Adults
425 East 25th Street
New York, NY 10010
(212) 481-4426
Primarily concerned with New York State laws, but can answer some questions on Federal laws.

Commission on Legal Problems of the Elderly
American Bar Association
1800 M Street NW, 2nd Floor, South Lobby
Washington, DC 20036
(202) 331-2297
Public education and awareness of legal issues affecting older persons.

Council of Better Business Bureaus
4200 Wilson Blvd.., 8th Floor
Arlington, VA 22205
(703) 276-0133
Sponsors consumer education and public information programs.

Legal Counsel for the Elderly
601 E Street, NW
Washington, DC 20049
(202) 434-2120
Through funding from AARP and other sources, this agency provides legal assistance on benefits eligibility, Social Security and other issues of special interest to older persons.

National Academy of Elder Law Attorneys
655 North Alvernon Way, Suite 108
Tucson, AZ 85711
(602) 881-4005
Provides listing of 400 member attorneys in the U.S. specializing in elder law. Cost is $25. Publishes Model Statement of Home Care Client Rights and Responsibilities *which benefits all users of home care.*

National Resources Center for Consumers of Legal Services
3254 Jones Court
Washington, DC 20007
(202) 338-0714

National Senior Citizens Law Center
1815 H Street, NW, Suite 700
Washington, DC 20006
(202) 887-5280
The NSCLC serves as a clearinghouse on legal issues concerning the elderly, addressing Social Security concerns, age discrimination, Medicare and Medicaid, nursing homes and consumer products. Individual clients are not accepted, but assistance is provided to lawyers and advocates.

Chapter Eight — Supervising Your Caregiver

Alcohol and Drug Abuse Clearinghouse
11426 Rockview Drive, Suite 200
Rockville, MO 20852
1-800-336-4797 or (301) 468-2600

American Association of Homes for the Aging
901 E Street NW, Suite 500
Washington, DC 20004-2837
(202) 783-2242
Publishes a brochure that discusses the range of home services that may be available. For a free copy of Community Services for Older People Living at Home, *send a self-addressed, legal-size, stamped envelope to the above address.*

Consumer Information Center
PO Box 100
Pueblo, CO 81009
Write for a listing of free government publications.

Foundation for Hospice and Homecare
519 C Street, NE, Stanton Park
Washington, DC 20002
(202) 547-6586
Ask for a list of accredited homemaker and home health aide services and information on how to select home and hospice services.

National Consumers League
815 15th Street NW, Suite 928
Washington, DC 20005
(202) 639-8140
For a single copy of All About Home Care: A Consumer's Guide, *send self-addressed, 55-cent stamped envelope. Order #4203. The League's* Primer on Long-Term Care *describes assisted living and many other types of long term care. To order, send a $4 check payable to the National Consumers League. Also available at $4 is* Consumer's Guide to Home Health Care, *which discusses all aspects of home health care.*

Chapter Nine — Finding and Using Community Resources

American Red Cross (National Headquarters)
430 18th Street, NW
Washington DC 20006
(202) 737-8300

American Society on Aging
833 Market Street, Suite 512
San Francisco, CA 94103
(415) 543-2617
A professional association that disseminates information on aging through publications, conferences and training events.

National Association of State Units on Aging
1225 I Street NW, Suite 725
Washington, DC 20005
(202) 898-2578
The state unit on aging is designed by the Governor to provide leadership and to develop comprehensive systems for elder persons throughout the state. (See Appendix F for further information.)

National Council on Aging, Inc.
Family Caregivers Program
409 3rd Street, S.W., Suite 200
Washington, DC 20024
(202) 479-1200
Provides information on services and programs in the field of aging. Disseminates information on a number of age-related issues. Write for Caregiving Kit, which includes six pamphlets. Cost is $6.00, including mailing charges.

National Council of Senior Citizens
1313 F Street, NW
Washington DC 2004-1171
(202) 347-8800
NCSC is one of America's largest membership organizations for the elderly. The Council publishes the Retirement Newsletter *to inform retirees about federal and state programs for elder people.*

National Hispanic Council on Aging
2713 Ontario Road, NW
Washington, DC 20008
(202) 265-1288
A non-profit, membership-based organization that promotes the well-being of Hispanic elderly.

National Institute on Aging
Public Information Center
Building 31, Room 5C27
9000 Rockville Pike
Bethesda MD 20892
1-800-222-2225
Provides a variety of publications on health and aging.

Chapter Ten — Dealing with Taxes, Insurance, and Laws

Service Corps of Retired Executives (SCORE)
409 3rd Street SW, 4th Floor
Washington, DC 20024
(202) 205-6762 or (800) 634-0245
A nonprofit association, sponsored by the Small Business Administration, that provides free business counseling. Look in the U.S. Government section in your phone book for the SCORE office that serves your area.

Social Security Administration
Office of Public Inquiries
6401 Security Boulevard
Balltimore MD 21235
(800) 772-1213
Provides information about Social Security, Medicare and Medicaid.

The Partnership Group, Inc.
840 West Main Street
Lansdale, PA 19446
1-800-VIP-KIDS/1-800-847-5437
A nationwide family resource service which provides referral and consultation on caregiving issues to business, government and industry.

U.S. Small Business Administration
Offices of Business Development
409 Third Street SW
Washington DC 20416
(202) 205-7000
Statewide network of resources available, addressing crime prevention, personnel management and other types of technical assistance.

Work/Family Elder Directions
930 Commonwealth Avenue
Boston, MA 92215-1212
(617) 566-1800
A nationwide resource that provides dependent care services to major corporations.

Chapter 11 — Agency-Directed Home Care

American Federation of Home Health Agencies
1320 Fenwick Lane, Suite 100
Silver Spring, Maryland 20910
(800) 368-5927
Trade association of Medicare-certified Home Health Care Agencies.

American Hospital Association
Division of Ambulatory and Home Care Services
840 North Lake Shore Drive
Chicago, Illinois 60611
(312) 280-6000
Trade association for hospitals.

Joint Commission on the Accreditation of Healthcare
Organizations
One Renaissance Boulevard
Oakbrook Terrace, IL 60181
Professional accreditation organization.

Visiting Nurse Associations of America
3801 East Florida Avenue, Suite 806
Denver, CO 80210
(303) 753-0218
Operates a toll-free referral line linking patients to local community Visiting Nurse Associations. For information regarding the VNA in your area call (800) 426-2547.

National Association for Home Care
519 C Street NE, Stanton Park
Washington, D.C. 20002-5809
(202) 547-7424
Accredits and approves homemaker/home care aide organizations. Publishes Handbook for the Home Health Aide, *a quick review of the specific skills required in homemaking and personal care ($8.95, plus $3.50 shipping). NAHC also produces several periodicals, including* Caring, *a monthly magazine, and* Home Care News, *a monthly newspaper.*

REVIEW TEAM MEMBERS

John A. Cutter is elder affairs reporter and parent care columnist for the *St. Petersburg Times* in Florida. He is the 1994 winner of the media award for regional/local reporters from the American Society of Aging, and has lectured on "Building Media Bridges" before the ASA, the Florida Council on Aging and other community groups. Mr. Cutter received a 1994 public awareness award from the Alzheimer's Association of Tampa Bay and also recently helped start the Journalists Exchange on Aging, a new national organization of reporters and writers who cover aging issues. He is a graduate of Fordham University in the Bronx, NY.

Louise Fradkin, M.L.S., is the co-founder of Children of Aging Parents (CAPS). She is the editor of the CAPS newsletter. For 21 years she was Head of Reference at Trenton State College in New Jersey. She has also worked as an architectural designer having received a B.A. in architecture from the University of Pennsylvania. Ms. Fradkin was a caregiver from 1974-1992 for her mother and her experiences as a bewildered caregiver led to her co-founding CAPS.

C. Elaine Jensen, M.A., is a gerontologist and a medical social worker with extensive clinical experience in working with patients, families and caregivers. She develops inservices and training programs for registered nurses and home-health aides, as well as stimulating community interest in aging issues through public speaking. She is a graduate of the University of South Florida.

Grace Lebow, a Diplomat in Clinical Social Work, is a co-founder and co-director of Aging Network Services, a national network of geriatric social workers since 1982. She was the Treatment Therapist on an NIH Research Grant titled, "Crisis Intervention in Dying and Bereavement," and was Director of Social Work at the Hebrew Home of Greater Washington. She brings to her private practice professional as well as personal experience with older people and their families. Mrs. Lebow received her degrees in Occupational Therapy from Tufts University in 1952 and Social Work from Simmons College in 1972.

Thomas W. Rezanka, J.D., is an Elder Law and Trusts & Estates attorney in Palm Harbor, Florida. He graduated from Stetson University College of Law in 1980. He is a member of the National Academy of Elder Law Attorneys, the Florida and American Bar Associations and the Clearwater Bar Association. Mr. Rezanka stresses in his practice the necessary preplanning to avoid guardianship and to afford nursing home care.

INDEX

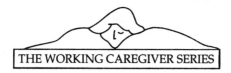
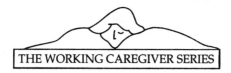
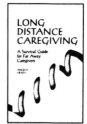
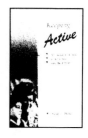
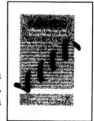
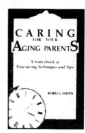